The No-Hysterectomy Option
Your Body–Your Choice

Herbert A. Goldfarb, MD FACOG, FACS

with

Judith Greif, MS, RNC, FNP

John Wiley & Sons, Inc.

New York • Chichester • Brisbane • Toronto • Singapore

This publication is designed to provide accurate and authoritative information in regard to the subject matter covered. It is sold with the understanding that the publisher and authors are not engaged in rendering medical or other professional service. If medical advice or other expert assistance is required, the services of a competent professional person should be sought. The names used for case histories are not patient's real names.

Library of Congress Cataloging-in-Publication Data

Goldfarb, Herbert A.
    The no-hysterectomy option: your body—your choice / by
Herbert A. Goldfarb with Judith Greif.
      p. cm.
    Includes bibliographical references (p. 227) and index.
    ISBN 0-471-53232-0 (c). -- ISBN 0-471-51615-5 (p)
    1. Hysterectomy. 2. Hysterectomy--Decision making. I. Greif,
Judith. II. Title.
RG391.G64 1990
618.1'453--dc20
                                     90-12692
                                          CIP

Printed in the United States of America
90 91 10 9 8 7 6 5 4 3 2 1

Dedication

To our families . . .

To Laurence, who inspired this idea and who taught me about giving one hundred and ten percent . . .

To Lisa, who soars beyond dreams . . .

To Scott, whose future is boundless . . .

To Beverly, who is the lighthouse of our lives . . .

H.G.

***

To Ruth, my sister and best friend, whom I respect tremendously for her courage, and whose success, wit, and wisdom I strive to emulate. Without you, this book would never have been a reality . . .

To my mother and father, in gratitude for the selfless generosity, patience, encouragement, guidance, love, and support that only nurturing parents can provide . . .

To Samantha, who was born a month after this book was born. You grew together . . .

And to Joe, my Don Quixote, who showed me that dreams are not impossible and that windmills fuel a love that is boundless.

J.G.

Preface

As to diseases, make a habit of two things; to help or at least not to harm.

—Hippocrates, 400 B.C.

According to recent statistics, in North America a hysterectomy is performed about once every 30 seconds. That's nearly one million hysterectomies per year! In fact, a woman stands a greater than 50 percent chance that she will undergo a hysterectomy by the time she approaches age 65. And, tragically, the surgery usually occurs at around age 35, when a woman is still in her reproductive years. Add to that the horrifying fact that over 2,000 women die from hysterectomies annually, with another 240,000 suffering major complications. The numbers become especially staggering in light of the evidence uncovered by numerous analyses of these procedures which conclude that *anywhere from 90 to 95 percent of these surgeries are elective!* Hysterectomy remains the most frequently performed major operation even though half the population (men) never require this surgery.

In their 1979 book, *Understanding Hysterectomy: A Woman's Guide,* Drs. Giustini and Keefer wrote:

> Most people have known someone who continues to bleed from the uterus no matter what the doctor tries. Flooding causing social embarrassment, or the necessity of wearing a pad two or more weeks monthly are problems for which women want solutions. Most doctors try hormone therapy or repeated D&Cs (scraping of the womb) to correct or control these troublesome complaints. After a woman has had three or more D&Cs, or has taken several courses of hormone therapy, the patient tires of the "conservative" approach. She wants something done. Hysterectomy is definitive, corrective, and permanent treatment. Often no abnormal tissue is found in the removal of the uterus, but clearly that did not mean the operation was unnecessary.

The opinions expressed by Giustini and Keefer in many ways reflect a mentality that pervaded the medical community a decade ago. In fairness, options *were* limited in 1979. Unfortunately, however, this mind-set is still with us today—the notion that a hysterectomy is a relatively risk-free panacea for the woman who is troubled by a gynecologic problem, has completed her family, and wants to eliminate the nuisance of menstruation. Nothing could be farther from the truth. All major surgery is fraught with complications. Hysterectomy is no exception, sometimes resulting in: hemorrhage, urinary tract trauma, intestinal injuries, posthysterectomy depression, sexual dysfunction, early ovarian failure, heart disease and osteoporosis.

This book is about changing this mentality and discovering options. It reexamines the propriety of hysterectomy and questions traditional medical practice. It challenges when hysterectomy is "indicated" versus when it is truly *necessary,* primarily from the woman's perspective, to safeguard her life or substantially improve its quality.

I remember back in the 1960s when my mother-in-law announced that she had just come from visiting her gynecologist. He told her that "it was time she had a hysterectomy." He said that her problems were minor, but that after a woman reaches age 40 she really "ought to" have a hysterectomy. "It would save a lot of troubles later on," he reassured her. Fortunately, her son-in-law advised her to the contrary.

We need to revise our thinking that hysterectomy is benign and convenient, and that there is no other hope for women faced with certain gynecologic problems. As we will see, hysterectomy is far from benign and there certainly is a great deal of hope and reason for optimism in terms of maintaining a woman's reproductive integrity.

Unlike the medical practitioners of the past, today we know that the uterus is more than a receptacle for the fetus. While we still do not completely comprehend the role of the uterus, this lack of understanding is not a valid reason for removing it. Yet hysterectomies are performed nearly one million times per year in North America. The cost of hysterectomy is too high—physically, emotionally, sexually, and economically—for us to stand idly by when there are options to having one's uterus removed.

Only in the last five years has the technology been born that allows us to present significant alternatives to routine hysterectomy, for persistent prolonged menstrual flow.

It is true that there are many women who have expressed no untoward after-effects as a result of a hysterectomy, but others have revealed significant depression over the removal of their uterus. The medical literature is replete with reports not only of physical complications, but of emotional problems developing after hysterectomy.

I came to realize that we had to calculate a risk/reward ratio to identify which patients would suffer from the performance of the procedure. The more I thought about this, the more I reasoned that one of the most important things that I could do was to help women stay healthy and intact and avoid frivolous hysterectomy at all cost.

In 1971, I was first exposed to the instrument called the hysteroscope, which allowed me to examine the cavity of the uterus at the time of a routine procedure, such as dilation and curettage. I was attending a course given by Dr. Robert Neuwirth, a true pioneer in the field. At that time, hospitals did not routinely offer hysteroscopes to their physicians, but I had such vision of the efficacy of being able to examine the entire cavity of the uterus (rather than perform a blind curettage procedure) that I purchased my own hysteroscope and proceeded to perform diagnostic hysteroscopies at no charge to my patients during those early years until I became proficient at the procedure.

In 1981, I became familiar with the work of Dr. Milton Goldrath in Detroit. Dr. Goldrath, in 1979, had established the first research protocol using the Neodynium Yttrium-aluminum garnet laser (ND:YAG or YAG for short) to treat women with uncontrollable uterine hemorrhage, and I knew that this symptom accounted for over 50 percent of all hysterectomies. Dr. Goldrath's impetus to perform this procedure was twofold. First, he was an expert hysteroscopist, involved in the art of examining the inside of the uterine cavity with a fiberoptic scope. Second, he had been familiar with this new YAG laser, which has as its major effect the ability to create depth of penetration and destruction of tissue at a depth greater than the initial zone of impact. Slowly, but surely, I began to realize that there was a possibility of making an impact in the treatment of abnormal uterine bleeding and the preservation of uterine function.

Instead of advocating hysterectomy, Dr. Goldrath was able to destroy the lining of the uterus (or endometrium) in patients who were too sick to undergo hysterectomy. He did this using minimal anesthesia, with a procedure that took less than an hour to perform and after which the patients were able to return home the same day.

In the early 1980s I began to read about the use of the laser in gynecological practice. I had often been frustrated during surgical procedures at my inability to perform operative procedures using endoscopes which I had come to rely on for diagnostic purposes. After hearing about the laser, I decided that this was a marvelous tool for operative endoscopy—operating through a scope. How wonderful it would be if we could cut, coagulate, and remove tissue through a scope without opening the abdominal cavity and without the threat of bleeding or the difficulties that electrocoagulations created.

In 1983, when I attended my first course in laser surgery, Dr. Milton Goldrath was one of the participants and teachers. In 1985 I was trained in carbon dioxide (CO_2) laser laparoscopy and was the first physician in New Jersey to use the technique. In 1986, I went to Chicago to learn the ND:YAG laser procedure that Dr. Goldrath was advocating, along with another pioneer, Dr. Frank Loffer of Phoenix, Arizona.

After the hysteroscopic YAG ablation procedure was given Food and Drug Administration clearance in 1986, I traveled to Detroit, Dr. Goldrath's home, and spent time with him on a one-to-one basis honing my skills. Six months later, I went back to see Dr. Goldrath with questions and problems concerning the proper performance of the procedure. Now I felt confident enough to attempt the procedure on my patients. In 1987, after selecting my first patient (with her permission and knowledge that this was a new technique) I performed the first ND:YAG procedure ever done in New Jersey and I am happy to report that it was successful.

Over the course of the last three years, an increasing number of physicians have attempted to learn the YAG laser technique. In 1987, I presented the first course in laser surgery at the New Jersey College of Medicine and Dentistry, which included the YAG laser endometrial ablation technique.

Now, in 1990, a recent letter from the American College of Obstetrics and Gynecology had stated that it is no longer considered an experimental procedure. So, we have come a long way in the last three years.

Other new techniques have allowed us to present significant alternatives to our patients. These include new hormonal therapies such as the GnRH agonist, which controls vaginal hemorrhage and reduces the size of uterine tumors. Myomectomy certainly offers an extremely palatable alternative to hysterectomy, and in combination with the use of the new GnRH agonist, we can reduce the size of myomas (fibroids) to the point where they can be easily removed with minimal blood loss.

We have also begun to remove certain uterine myomas through the vagina. Whether by grasping, lasering, or using the urologic resectoscope, we can now resculpture the uterine cavity and reduce or eliminate abnormal bleeding. These and other techniques will be explained more fully as we go into the text.

The use of the CO_2 laser through the laparoscope has allowed us to treat women with endometriosis and avoid open abdominal laparotomy, as well as hysterectomy.

Finally, the treatment of the uterine cervix with the CO_2 laser allows us to destroy premalignant conditions, such as dysplasia (abnormal growth) and human papilloma virus (condylomata), which may, if left untreated, progress to become cervical cancer.

Unfortunately, we cannot prevent every hysterectomy. Certain uterine myomas may have grown grotesquely large with severe forms of hemorrhage, and may be too late for us to reverse. However, we now posses a much better understanding of what happens to women when they have a hysterectomy and we have much improved modalities for coping with the physical and emotional devastation that often follows hysterectomy.

Utilizing the techniques that I have described, namely, hormonal therapy, myomectomy, laser surgery, and careful observation, we may be able to eliminate as many as one-half to two-thirds of the hysterectomies performed each year.

One of the real problems in making an impact on the hysterectomy statistics is that there are relatively few gynecologists trained in these advanced techniques.

I have been participating in educational programs and laser courses since 1987 but there are well over 28,000 obstetrician-gynecologists practicing in the United States today, and only 15 to 25 physicians can be trained at a time using laboratory and lecture techniques, so we have a long way to go in making a significant dent in reducing the number of hysterectomies performed.

The motivation that will be required to push physicians into updating their knowledge will revolve around public outcry and the consumer demand for alternatives to hysterectomy. As must be obvious, the cost of laser equipment is stratospheric. Each laser sells for somewhere between $60,000 and $100,000. Therefore, if physicians are to make use of this technology, there must be enough of them trained in these new techniques to make it economically feasible for hospitals to invest money in laser technology. As more consumer groups bring mounting pressure to bear upon physicians to provide alternative treatments, administrators will get the word and physicians will see the handwriting on the wall.

Before I was born, I had a sister whom I will never know, because in those days before routine use of antibiotics, she died of sepsis following a so-called routine tonsillectomy. My mother went on to have two sons, and while she obviously loves us, she frequently laments the loss of her only daughter. Her daughter was taken from her unnecessarily at a time when tonsillectomy was common. We now know the importance of tonsils to the immune system, and the dangers of unwarranted operations. Perhaps her death was not in vain because through my deeply personal and tragic experience, I have become particularly sensitized to this cavalier outlook with respect to surgery. Hundreds or thousands of women are told each year that a hysterectomy is necessary. Perhaps you or a loved one will be among those people who have been or will be offered hysterectomy as a panacea for your gynecological problems. It is for you that I am writing this book. While we do not have all of the answers yet, I hope I will stimulate you to ask the right questions and help you to make the best, most informed decision for yourself. It is my fervent hope that this book will make an impact in helping women to avoid unnecessary hysterectomy.

Montclair, New Jersey
1990

Postscript

When I first undertook this project, the main thrust of this book was telling women how and why to avoid hysterectomies. However, as I became more involved in its research and writing, I realized that there is much more to say. As a result, this book has taken on a much broader perspective, although its central focus remains hysterectomy. It has become a book about the physical and psychological aspects of women's health. It is an attempt at a thorough discussion encompassing all of the principal conditions which can and have resulted in major abdominal surgery for women. It discusses in detail what these conditions are, how they have been diagnosed and treated in the past, as well as what new and future therapies are becoming available. The new therapies I have recommended take into consideration the total woman, not merely her pelvic organs. It is my aim to help a woman to deal with a serious medical problem equipped with maximal knowledge and understanding so that she can make a truly informed decision regarding its management. It is my strong conviction that a woman should be a partner in her care with her physician and not just a passive recipient.

Years ago, when a pregnant woman went into labor she was placed flat on her back and given a pharmacopeia of pain and "twilight sleep" preparations to sedate her until it was finally time to whisk her off to the delivery room. There, she'd be strapped down, placed under general anesthesia, and her baby delivered while an anxious father paced the hallways. The baby would be routinely injected with narcan to reverse its narcotic stupor and moved into the nursery. Later, the mother could "visit" her baby, but only during specified hours. Today, women are up walking until active labor begins. If they wish to be, mothers are fully alert and unmedicated throughout the birth of their children, which now takes place in homelike birthing rooms. Fathers are encouraged to participate in their wives' labor and to be present during the delivery. In effect, women no longer unquestioningly accept or even tolerate the passive role to which they were delegated during childbirth a generation ago. As a result, obstetrical philosophy and practice has changed dramatically. Now it is time for gynecology to follow suit.

However, this book goes beyond helping women to understand more about their bodies and demand more of their physicians for the sake of avoiding major surgery alone. It is also about minimizing the impact of a chronic condition on a woman's lifestyle so that she can avoid major upheavals in her career and in her personal life.

During the Victorian Era, the weak and wan female was a popular image. Perhaps because they posed a threat to their male contemporaries, intelligent and active women might be told that they suffered from hysteria or so-called neurasthenia and that they must take a "rest cure." This involved taking to one's bed for weeks or even months during which time the woman couldn't read, write, or enjoy any social contact. That this alleged "cure" could actually itself induce madness is documented in one account by a noted feminist of the time, Charlotte Perkins Gilman, who wrote a famous story about her experience, recently dramatized on PBS, called, *The Yellow Wallpaper.*

Women no longer desire or tolerate prolonged idle periods of recuperation. In addition, they expect to play an active role in maintaining or restoring their health. To meet these goals, this book discusses nutrition, exercise, and psychotherapy in terms of what you can do to keep mind and body sound whether you are attempting to avoid hysterectomy or cope with its aftermath.

Acknowledgments

A great many people, including friends, family members and colleagues were indispensible in supporting us through this undertaking. They served as resources and sounding boards, as well as offered time, advice, encouragement, and moral support. To them we are greatly indebted.

This book involved a tremendous amount of research. We would especially like to thank the staff of the Health Sciences Library Tishman Learning Center, Montefiore Medical Center, Bronx, New York for assisting in this task. In particular, Josie Lim, Deborah Green, and Vernon Bruette were unwavering sources of assistance and information. In addition, Ann Marie Palladino is to be thanked for facilitating a computer search of the literature that saved hours of tedious manual work.

For assistance in preparing the manuscript, including proofreading, editing, and photocopying, the authors wish to acknowledge Joseph Pedreiro—a seasoned professional in these and other tasks.

Our gratitude is extended to Rachel Feldblum for her helpful professional guidance in the section concerning emotional issues related to hysterectomy.

Finally, we would like to commend and acknowledge the staff at John Wiley and Sons, especially David Sobel, Ruth Greif, and Ted Scheffler for their invaluable assistance in making this book the best it could be.

Special Acknowledgments

I wish to acknowledge the influences on my life that gave me the courage to tread on hallowed ground . . .

- My teachers at New York University College of Medicine, who taught me not to compromise excellence
- Sophie Kleegman, M.D., wherever she may be—at least one person listened

- Richard Berman, M.D., my longtime friend, who encouraged me never to accept mediocrity
- Charles Debrovner, M.D., whose friendship of 30 years has been cherished, and whose honesty and strength of character and achievement have been an inspiration
- Milton Goldrath, M.D., who had patience and time for me
- Franklin Loffer, M.D., whose kindness and excellence were a source of unbelievable help
- The staff at Montclair Community Hospital, who have endured my desire to do better
- Irene Newton, R.N., my friend and nurse for over 20 years who has given so much for so long
- Anthony Oropollo, M.D., for having the faith to listen and to support me when I needed him the most
- Emily Murphy, for being there with an open door and open ear, and having the courage to see the light
- Judith Greif, R.N.C., who was incredibly competent, and who I really came to admire and respect during our time together
- Stanley Goldfarb, M.D., who has set an example of excellence and showed me that it could be done
- My mother, whose persistence and strength of character gave me the will to go on. Her love and support has never wavered
- My father, wherever he may be, whose life was a textbook of determination and character. I wish you were here to read this book

—Herbert Goldfarb, M.D.

Contents

Part 1

The Controversy

By eight o'clock we were in the operating room. Once in the OR, how did I feel? I felt important. . . . There is something about a uniform, too, that makes one feel important. My whole being reeked of my station. I was an insider. I looked just like the others. I had a place, a job, and I was being taught the secrets of medicine. If we had expressed our feelings of elitism, we might have said, "How terrible never to see the inside of the OR, never to have a role in the drama there." I was ashamed of the power I felt in that room, ashamed of what I was becoming, and yet I was also enjoying it.

—Michelle Harrison, M.D.
A Woman In Residence

1

About the Controversy: Do You Really Need a Hysterectomy?

If like all human beings, he [the gynecologist] is made in the image of the Almighty, and he is kind, then his kindness and concern for his patient may provide her with a glimpse of God's image.

—Russell C. Scott, M.D.

The Historical Perspective

In Dr. Evans' book, *How to Keep Well*, the author explains the cure for syphilis, which may be contracted through the use of an "unclean towel" or "toilet." He recommends, "one injection of neosalvarsan . . . followed by six months of mercury injections . . . three more injections of neosalvarsan . . . followed by [two additional years of] mercury injected twice each week . . . [and] mercury by mouth." We now know, of course, that penicillin is the cure for syphilis. Worse still, excess intake of mercury can lead to insanity ("Mad Hatter's Disease") and even death. Here, then, is one case in point where the cure was as bad, if not worse, than the disease.

Obviously, medicine is an ever-evolving science, where practices and opinions as to what may be "necessary and indicated" for a particular disease process change with the times. This chapter is about the history of women's health, the evolution of women's surgery, and how they have led to the trends and controversies we see today concerning hysterectomy.

According to Robert Pokras and Vicki Hufnagel, two researchers who analyzed data for the National Health Survey, as recently as 1980, hysterectomy was the most frequently performed major surgery, outdistancing tonsilectomy, cholecystectomy (removal of the gallbladder), hernia repair, coronary bypass procedures—even cesarean section. It is also one of the most ancient of surgeries. The Greek physician Archigenes was said to have performed hysterectomy in Rome in the first century A.D. And, ironically enough, unlike most other things in Western medicine (such as the treatment of syphilis alluded to before), hysterectomy has remained relatively unchanged throughout nearly two millennia.

The first obstetrician-gynecologists were the women priestess/healers of Ancient Sumer, Assyria, Egypt, and Greece who attended the births of the women of those cultures. Throughout the Middle Ages, the Renaissance, and up to the Industrial Age, obstetrics, through the practice of midwifery, remained the exclusive domain of the female practitioner.

Men, at the same time, were training as physicians and were gaining firsthand knowledge of internal anatomy and physiology. This initially came about with the embalmers of Ancient Egypt, 2300 years before the birth of Christ. The ancient Egyptians believed that life was a preparation for the afterlife, and that the embalmed body housed the eternal soul. They therefore carefully removed and preserved the liver, lungs, stomach, and intestines because these would be needed by the individual in the hereafter. In addition they removed the brain, bathing the skull with spices. They then carefully soaked and wrapped the remainder of the body with linens.

While the embalmers of Ancient Egypt were the first members of a civilization to examine internal anatomy and to try to explain physiology, they overlooked or misunderstood much of the significance of what they saw. The Egyptians believed that the body parts were linked to deities and that these organs together comprised a system of channels with the heart at its center. This was probably because they were cognizant of its pulsations throughout the body.

Small steps forward were made during the times of Hippocrates and Galen. Then, during the third century B.C., in Alexandria, Herophilus of Chalcedon, the Father of Anatomy and Erasistratus of Chios, the Father of Physiology became the first individuals to systematically and deliberately perform human dissections, thus significantly advancing our knowledge of the human body. Religious mandates against such practices came into effect soon after, and remained in place for centuries, stemming the advancing tides of medicine and surgery for many generations.

Medicine, as learned in universities by male physicians during the Middle Ages, was intimately tied to religion. Midwifery, however, became the stuff of superstition—literally "old wives'" tales—even witchcraft, which was evil and demonic.

These notions paved the way for male physicians to become involved, for the first time, in obstetrics, and, by association, gynecology. However, this practice was *not* condoned by many in the medical field. In her book, *Men Who Control Women's Health,* author Diane Scully quotes Dr. Samuel Gregory as writing, around 1848, to implore physicians to abandon midwifery, because,

> . . . the introduction of men into the lying-in chamber, in place of female attendants, has increased the suffering and dangers of childbearing women, and brought multiplied injuries and fatalities upon mothers and children; it violates the sensitive feelings of husbands and wives, and causes an untold amount of domestic misery; the unlimited intimacy between a numerous profession and the female population silently and effectually wears away female delicacy and professional morality, and tends, probably more than any other cause in existence, to undermine the foundation of public virtue.

Sadly, medical and social practices of the mid-1800s made this true. Early nineteenth-century physicians lacked knowledge of anesthesia and antibiotics, worked with primitive instruments, and until Dr. Ignaz Semmelweis, often went from the autopsy room to the bed chamber without washing their equipment or their hands. As a result, unlike the midwives who were not involved in dissections of corpses, physicians themselves often spread death and disease from household to household by serving as the vehicle through which bacteria were transmitted.

Dr. Semmelweis significantly reduced the mortality rate from "childbed fever" by forcing the physicians on his staff at the Lying In Hospital in Vienna to wash with soap, water, and chlorine before entering the ward and before examining each patient. Instead of being hailed as a medical genius and dying triumphant, Dr. Semmelweis was chastised and condemned by his narrow-minded peers. He was driven to madness and died in an insane asylum of a blood infection, much like the women he had tried to save.

Victorian morals also precluded complete and proper examinations of female genitalia. During the 1800s, it was considered inappropriate and unscrupulous for male physicians to examine women, except by reaching up under their skirts while averting their eyes! This practice continued in some circles even after the invention of the speculum. Critics of this device, like Dr. Robert Brudenell Carter, argued vigorously against its use because he claimed to have seen "young, unmarried women of the middle class of society, reduced by the constant use of the speculum to the mental and moral condition of prostitutes."

And the delicacy, innocence, and "asexuality" of women during this time was to be preserved at all costs. Again, in 1848, Dr. Charles Meigs wrote, "I am proud to say . . . that there are women who prefer to suffer the extremity of danger and pain rather than waive those scruples of delicacy which prevent their maladies from being fully explored."

Before the nineteenth century, female sexuality was never acknowledged to be important, unique, or worthy of study. In the 1800s, for the first time, female sexuality became a subject, not merely of interest, but of substantial fear and loathing. As a result of this, women now ran the risk of having their lives placed in jeopardy from operative practices stemming from the need of male physicians to intervene. It was during this time that hysterectomy and oophorectomy (removal of the ovary) first came into vogue as the cure for nearly everything ailing the female, including: headaches, epilepsy, indigestion, backaches, liver trouble, and, of course, "excessive sexual desire."

The contradictory attitudes of society in general, and male physicians in particular, during this era are reflected in conflicting opinions regarding the preservation of the uterus. To some physicians, the female was viewed in the almost revered role of childbearer. One doctor even went so far as to say that the "the Almighty, in creating the female sex, had taken a uterus and built up a woman around it." Furthermore, society had a definite vested interest in keeping her a wife and mother. One well-documented example concerned the controversy surrounding whether Harvard should become coeducational. In 1873, Dr. Edward H. Clarke, a physician and Harvard professor, cautioned against a college education for women, as it would cause "uterine atrophy." Women were socialized to be docile, feeble, and subservient to men. If they were not, that's when medicine had to intervene, and despite their importance to the sanctity of childbearing, the female organs must be sacrificed.

From Hippocrates, who said, "What is Woman? Disease" to Freud, who contended that women were inferior creatures suffering from penis envy, castration complexes, and a host of neuroses, the unique physiology and psychology of women have often been misunderstood. This has often led to surgical excesses, especially during the nineteenth century. Dr. J. Marion Sims, a prominent name in gynecology even to this day, operated on slave women, repeatedly, without the use of anesthesia and without their consent, to perfect his cure for vesicovaginal fistula, a communication between the bladder and vagina usually as a result of birth trauma. Others performed clitoridectomies as a "cure" for nymphomania and masturbation. However, the ovary took the greatest abuse.

In *Understanding Hysterectomy*, Drs. Giustini and Keefer recount the story of a "daring young doctor," Kentucky surgeon Dr. Ephraim McDowell, who, in 1809, "without the benefit of anesthesia and sterile technique" is credited with performing the first oophorectomy, removing an ovarian tumor in a middle-aged woman. One has to wonder in this situation exactly who was the "daring" one— the doctor or *the patient!* But the onslaught was not to begin in earnest for another 40 years when a dentist in Massachusetts, named William T. G. Morton, demonstrated the use of ether to anesthetize a patient in order to remove a tumor on his neck. Now that women could be put to sleep, it was literally "open season" on the female internal organs. From the middle or late 1800s until as recently as the 1940s, thousands of women had their ovaries sacrificed, frequently for trivial and irrelevant reasons (i.e., overeating, disagreeable personalities, or lustful tendencies), and frequently at the cost of their lives. Martin Pernick, in *A Calculus of Suffering*, estimates that, prior to 1846 (the year anesthesia was introduced by Morton), perhaps 100 oophorectomies had been performed throughout the history of medicine. Then, from 1846 to 1878, a single physician, Dr. William Atlee, took out the ovaries of nearly 400 women. The champion of the oophorectomy movement was a surgeon from Georgia named Robert Battey who believed that through removal of the ovaries, one could control a woman's personality. Like Battey, Dr. David Gilliam boasted that, after oophorectomy, his patients were "tractable, orderly, industrious and cleanly." When some of their colleagues, such as Elizabeth Blackwell, America's first female doctor, balked, these gynecologists argued that insane women—having, of course, gotten that way from their wayward ovaries—had, in the words of Dr. William Goodell, no defense against undergoing the surgery:

> For, in the first place, an insane woman is no more a member of the body-politic, than a criminal; secondly, her death is always a relief to her dearest friends; thirdly, even in case of her recovery from mental disease, she is liable to transmit the taint of insanity to her children and to her children's children for many generations. . . .

Because it seemed in their minds to be more directly linked to a woman's ability to bear children, the battle for removal of the uterus was longer and more difficult. Ultimately, however, hysterectomy took root as the solution for that evil "curse" of the female form: menstruation. From earliest times, philosophers like Aristotle and Pliny the Elder warned of menstruating women—that they could cause wine to sour, crops to die—that their very look could cause an innocent person to become bewitched. And, of course, the very word "hysteria" comes to us from the Greek term for uterus, because, it was believed, insanity derived from a "wandering" of this organ. Menstruation was thought of as a monthly bloodletting whereby the body would rid itself of its poisons and excrements, automatically rendering women weak and inferior creatures. They were therefore obviously incapable of playing an equal role in society, and maybe, just maybe, they were even a little mad. (Vestiges of this are present today in some of the hype over "premenstrual syndrome.") Therefore, wouldn't a woman be "better off" without her uterus? Believe it or not, this notion lingers even today. While women began being literally castrated in significant numbers over a century ago, those times do not match up in volume to today's times when our "enlightened civilization" continues to practice hysterectomy and oophorectomy with astounding frequency.

The Modern Dilemma

In the days when I first trained and began to practice as a gynecologist, both physicians and the general public viewed hysterectomy as a benign procedure—even a welcome one. There is no question that the statistics in 1965, with regard to anesthesia, antibiotics, and blood replacement were certainly an improvement over those of the 1940s or even 1950s. We had better monitoring devices, better analgesics, and the public, in general, viewed surgery as something that was restorative rather than destructive. Many women felt that they would be better off for having their uterus removed, wouldn't have to worry about the monthly menstrual soaking, could avoid the concern of cancer and could take hormones and be young and feminine forever. Medicine and science had finally "solved" most of our problems.

The following passages are from a women's health-care book and a popular gynecological text, respectively—both written within the past 10 to 15 years, and both touting the miracle of hysterectomy.

Nancy Roeske in *The Woman Patient* cites a small study performed on women after they had undergone a hysterectomy in which she seems to imply that the procedure is a feminist and career woman's dream. Now women do not have to fear that either children or their troublesome uteri will interfere with their jobs and hobbies:

> The spontaneous expression of feeling "better than ever" and "glad to get it over with," as well as the relief from fear of pregnancy, enabled the woman to invest herself in, and find gratification from, her vocational and avocational interests. For these women, the uterus was no longer as highly valued as during their childbearing years. They had other sources for self-esteem which had, in the past, been sometimes limited by child care and the internal sexual organs' pathology. . . .

The author of the study goes on to admit, however, that these women experienced fatigue, constipation, gastritis, hot flashes, insomnia and "mourning" for up to a year postoperatively, but that these symptoms were "not incapacitating."

Even more dramatic are the statements made in Novak, Jones, and Jones' *Novak's Textbook of Gynecology* calling the uterus a "worthless organ" once childbearing is completed, and best eliminated because worse than being worthless, the uterus was the source of the menses:

> . . . menstruation is a nuisance to most women, and if this can be abolished . . . it would probably be a blessing to not only the women *but to their husbands.* . . . [emphasis added]

Taking this mind-set one step further, under no circumstances should one hesitate to perform a hysterectomy on postmenopausal women, whether that menopause had occurred naturally, or had been accomplished surgically. State Giustini and Keefer:

> She is no longer capable of becoming pregnant. The life-giving function of the uterus and ovaries has stopped. From this point on, there is no known value or function of the uterus. The ovaries, on the other hand, continue to function with decreasing hormone production, a fact that is considered by most American gynecologists to be of little value to the patient from a standpoint of good health and well being. . . .
>
> It is well accepted that when both ovaries are removed the uterus should be removed; only in exceptional circumstances should this organ be left in. The reason is a simple one—when both ovaries have been removed, the uterus becomes a functionless organ. The patient will not menstruate through it, and she will not be able to bear children with it. When one considers the risk of developing cancer in this now-useless organ, it is obvious why it is best removed.

As we shall see, the uterus and ovaries continue to be vital to women, beyond childbearing, beyond menopause, and beyond their purely reproductive functions. But these views were not so widely held in the mid-1960s. Rather, the fear of cancer was overwhelming. Unfortunately, physicians capitalized, perhaps unwittingly, on this all-pervasive fear. Small fibroid tumors were considered potentially dangerous and literally millions of hysterectomies were performed over the last 20 years with the diagnosis of rapidly enlarging fibroid tumors. Many of these tumors had grown from walnut to plum size and were the rationale for the hysterectomy. Uterine relaxation or prolapse was one of the frequent diagnoses that was used to justify hysterectomy and with the advent of insurance plans and the increasing utilization by patients and their physicians, surgery was now more affordable than ever. Another impetus to the growing number of hysterectomies was the sterilization committee that ruled on the proper requirements for sterilization. Depending on the patient's age, she might be required to have as many as 4, 5, or even 6 children before she would pass the criteria to be allowed sterilization. And remember, it was not until 1965 that the birth control pill came into general usage and, of course, abortion was illegal, so sterilization was a significant method of contraception in the 1950s and early 1960s.

Many physicians circumvented these rules by performing hysterectomies. In 1975, the American College of Obstetrician-Gynecologists estimated that 20 percent of hysterectomies were performed solely for sterilization purposes. Nationwide, hysterectomy rates rose precipitously.

Certain physicians didn't even draw the line at sterilization on demand by women. These physicians might determine sterilization to be "necessary" in certain extenuating circumstances. Again, we quote from Giustini and Keefer:

> Sterilization is a most controversial reason for a hysterectomy, but some circumstances might warrant the operation . . . an indication for the removal of a normal uterus [is] the case of the young woman with mental retardation. Here the uterus would be removed for two reasons: the elimination of menstrual periods, and to accomplish sterilization.
>
> A menstrual period can be a very traumatic event for a mentally retarded female. She does not understand the blood loss and she may not be able to cope with it. Also, the mentally retarded child can easily be the victim of unscrupulous sex offenders. A consequent pregnancy is an extremely serious situation.

One can only imagine how the authors would rate the physical and emotional trauma of major abdominal surgery (with the fear of hospitalization and the associated post-operative pain during the six-week recovery period) compared with the "trauma" of menses. Nor can one comprehend how having a hysterectomy prevents or even minimizes sexual abuse.

Be that as it may, often surgeons "did women a favor" by justifying to the tissue committees the indications for hysterectomy. Even though my colleagues were well aware that the procedures were being done for sterilization, I can personally recall numerous incidents when I had offered women the opportunity to have a hysterectomy for sterilization, under the guise of uterine relaxation, vaginal prolapse, or recurrent abdominal bleeding. When I look back over those days, I realize that even though we were trying to help our patients, in the long run, we probably did more harm than good.

I can vividly remember a patient who in 1970, only a few years after I had entered practice, desperately desired sterilization. She had two children. On examination, I noted that she had some uterine relaxation and she had a history of irregular vaginal bleeding. I offered her a vaginal hysterectomy and vaginal tightening. The vaginal tissues were cinched and the uterus was removed and the bladder was supported. The surgical procedure went quickly and smoothly and there were no apparent problems.

Shortly after we entered the recovery room, I noted that the patient was breathing with significant difficulty and there were small bubbles of fluid coming out of her mouth. I listened to her chest and immediately made the diagnosis of pulmonary edema (fluid in the lungs), usually a result of heart failure and probably brought on by poor oxygen supply during surgery. This perfectly healthy 40-year-old woman, who entered the hospital for an elective surgical procedure, was now at risk for her life. Emergency measures were taken, which included placing a tube in her windpipe, giving her oxygen, as well as drugs to strengthen the force of her heart, and diuretics to relieve any fluid overload, which reversed the condition.

I remember turning away from the patient after the emergency measures were undertaken and saying to myself, "what a close call." It was then I began to question, was this worth it? Was it worth exposing this woman to mortal danger for a procedure that was not absolutely necessary? Today fortunately, anesthesia is much improved. We have constant oxygen monitoring; we intubate all patients during major surgery. Nevertheless, one hears of sporadic episodes of healthy, young men and woman entering the hospital for a "benign" surgical condition and then of their untimely demise. I always think to myself the common bromide, the best safety device is a careful driver. Maybe the best safety device is to drive only when you must. Unfortunately, that was not the first time that disaster had struck.

I remember another situation when I was a resident on a rotation at a city hospital. It was a gray, dark winter's morning, when I left my apartment and traveled to a hospital in Harlem to begin a day's work in gynecological surgery. I was only a second-year gynecology resident; really just learning. Two of us were on rotation and had a well-known gynecologist attending physician who supervised our work. I climbed the three flights of stairs to the gynecological ward to see patients that I had operated on the day before. As I made my rapid rounds, one patient seemed to be sleeping. I chose not to wake her thinking that I would come back later and make more complete rounds. I went down to the operating room to begin the day's surgery. Just before the operation was to begin, I received an emergency phone call from the gynecology floor. The nurses had gone on their rounds taking blood pressure and pulse and the patient, whom I thought was sleeping, was not sleeping at all. She was dead. Somehow this woman had died in her sleep during the course of the night and no one had known. An autopsy was performed and it was noted that the site of surgery was completely normal. Something had obviously happened that we were not aware of and I never did find out why this woman died.

Here we had an apparently healthy woman who came to the hospital for a vaginal hysterectomy and repair for prolapse, perhaps also for sterilization, I don't recall exactly, and she died in her sleep—no one was even aware that there was a problem. I was deeply shaken and at this early stage of my career, I realized that not every surgical procedure ended happily and uneventfully.

As I look back over those days and the trauma, I am amazed at what we went through to learn to become physicians; but maybe I should say, it's astounding what our patients went through for us to become physicians. One point that keeps pounding at me repeatedly is, "I don't think we were ever totally imbued with the awesome responsibility that we had to protect our patients." I certainly was never adequately impressed by what it meant to be responsible for someone's life.

Actually, there was one person who, more than any other, set her own standards for medicine—standards perhaps one level above everyone else that I came into contact with. That physician, a pioneer in her own right, was Dr. Sophia Kleegman. Dr. Kleegman deserves a great deal of credit for sowing the seeds of doubt in my mind as to the wisdom of the procedures that we performed. She was kind; she related to me as a physician, and I spent a lot of time following her around the clinics at Bellevue learning from her insights and appreciating her compassion and sensitivity for her patients. She became a reproductive specialist when that was a rarity. Many of the residents did not take her seriously because she was so kind and homey; however, her patients took her seriously. Other gynecologists would send her patients with a type of chronic vaginal infection, called trichomonas, because she had a way of spending a great deal of time with patients and instructing them on hygiene and trying to help them overcome this problem. Today we have a medication, Flagyl, a very specialized antibiotic, that eliminates these infections in one to two days, but Dr. Kleegman taught me never to give up on a patient and to make every effort to deal with her problem. She also showed me that the standard approach to a medical problem is not always the correct one.

In fact, Dr. Kleegman was really the first teacher to show me that just caring for a patient with expectant observation, what some call "doing nothing," can be the best medicine. She had a very large practice and many of her patients had fibroid tumors, but often she would just examine and monitor and not operate. In fact, many of the young physicians jokingly referred to these patients as Dr. Kleegman's garden of fibroids. Most other physicians would have done hysterectomies and profited greatly from this garden, but Dr. Kleegman was different. She merely treated these patients with tender loving care, saw them once every six months to a year and as long as their symptoms were not terribly significant, she kept them from the clutches of the surgeon.

I must admit that I did not always follow Dr. Kleegman's dictum of expectant observation. It was certainly easy to get on the bandwagon to perform the surgical procedure that we were taught was "our operation" and start to think about how many hysterectomies we could do. Over the years, the trauma that my patients have faced, and my own introspection, has gradually taught me to appreciate the wisdom of her thinking, and to finally come to the realization that sometimes the best thing we can do for a patient is to *do nothing*.

One of my real causes célèbre is to talk about the terms "indicated" versus "necessary." How in the old days we used to justify hysterectomy by citing "indications" such as a growing fibroid or recurrent vaginal bleeding. Whether these symptoms were excessive or not, whether it was the last straw or not, we tried to convince our patients that hysterectomy was the best option that could solve the problem—we could cut out the disease. There would be no change in their bodies or their minds. They would only be healthier for what we were able to do for them! We began to believe our own hype that the presence of this tumor was some evil situation and that we were best off by removing the uterus. Why would anyone want to leave a fibroid uterus in a woman in her 40s when the tumor could be removed? We were all wrong. How could we have known that this mind-set would cost lives, lead to unnecessary suffering and pain, and would not really improve the quality of most patients' lives. Therefore, when you hear the term, "the surgery is indicated," remember the axiom—"is it indicated or is it necessary"? I believe strongly now that surgery should not be performed unless it will significantly change the quality of life, unless it is the only proper course of action, unless the alternatives require that it be performed.

For example, ovarian tumors are potentially dangerous. They are often silent killers. No one in their right mind would leave a persistent ovarian tumor without recommending surgery. Cancer of the uterus or cervix is a potentially lethal condition if untreated. Nevertheless, fibroids are 99.5 percent benign. Therefore, they fall into a different category and my plea for conservatism, for doing everything in our power to avoid the radical approach of hysterectomy with its attendant complications, its psychological destructiveness, is certainly worthwhile to heed. *Saving or greatly improving the quality of a woman's life is the only true indication for surgery.*

Indicated or Necessary?

While it probably began in the 1940s, the debate concerning necessary versus unnecessary hysterectomy really heated up about 20 years ago. That was when certain physicians and researchers began to notice some very disturbing trends in the statistics on hysterectomy. The most basic and alarming of these was the escalation in the numbers of procedures being performed. They noted that, from 1965 to 1975, the annual numbers of hysterectomies had spiraled upward from 427,000 to 725,000. (After peaking in 1975, it gradually tapered off to a fairly steady rate of between 650,000 and 675,000 per year. In 1987, the most recent year for which data is available, there were 655,000 of these surgeries in the United States.) Women now had about a 62 percent chance that they would undergo hysterectomy in their lifetime. Like a cancer, surgical procedures were multiplying at a rate that was four times the growth rate of the population.

Of crucial interest to these researchers was the fact that the growing numbers of hysterectomy were totally unrelated to any coinciding growth in the amount of pathology in women. If women weren't any more diseased, what, then, was the cause of all of these hysterectomies?

Writing in the *New England Journal of Medicine* in 1979, Dr. John Bunker exposed some astonishing new data. There were twice as many surgeons in the United States in proportion to the overall population as in England and Wales, and they performed twice as many operations. Specifically hysterectomy was shown to be even more excessive, with relative rates of 213 per 100,000 in the British Isles as compared with 516 per 100,000 in the United States. He cited "socioeconomic, organizational, philosophical, geographical, and population differences," *but could find no medical reasons,* to account for the discrepancy. In other words, according to Dr. Bunker, the British system of socialized medicine had inherent safeguards and lacked incentives for surgery that differed from the American fee-for-service system.

By the 1970s, many Americans had health insurance plans which allowed them to afford the "luxury" of "elective" surgery. They could simply go to their doctor, sometimes a general practitioner, who would recommend and perform their operation without a second opinion being called for. In England, however, surgeons practiced out of hospitals, not in solo settings, and relied on referrals from general practitioners or internists to build their caseload. Rather than being the gatekeeper, they were the consultant—the end of the line. And with socialized medicine, there was no financial gain in doing vast numbers of operations.

Finally, said Dr. Bunker, there seemed to be a fundamental philosophical difference between the U.S. surgeon's attitude toward what operating could accomplish as compared with the British. American doctors, said Dr. Bunker, were "more aggressive" and held "higher expectations." That American doctors derive great satisfaction from performing surgery seems to be supported by the research done by Diane Scully. She interviewed obstetrician-gynecologists in training at New England hospitals. Nothing can illustrate the attitudes of eager new surgeons better than this passage from her interview with one young doctor:

> You open the belly . . . you take something out, and the patient gets better . . . I don't know, it is the same thing as in kindergarten when

you took a little car apart. . . . The thing with surgery is that you have
something to show. You have a headache and I give you an aspirin
and it goes away, fine. If you have postpartum bleeding and you need
a hysterectomy and I take out your uterus and everything is fine, you
can say, "look at that fine piece of surgery I did.

How doctors are educated, and the philosophies instilled in them
by the standards of the community where they practice, seem to
play a key role in how they approach surgery. Consider the results
of an extensive study published in *Scientific American* by Wennberg
and Gittelsohn a few years after Dr. Bunker's. Surprisingly, the
authors found that "the amount and cost of hospital treatment
[including surgery] in a community have more to do with the
numbers of physicians there, their medical specialties, and the
procedures they prefer than with the health of the residents." They
discussed an almost unbelievable example of two cities in Maine
less than 20 miles apart. In the first city, hysterectomy was done so
frequently that if the rate were to persist, *70 percent of the women there
would have had a hysterectomy by the time they were 70 years of age!* In the
second city, only 25 percent would have. In examining the health
of the two groups of women residing in each city, they found no
differences. Neither could they explain this phenomenon via a
difference in their wealth, insurance coverage, nor even, in this
case, the numbers of physicians or hospital beds. It seemed the
sole difference between these two communities was in the style of
medical practice—one city's doctors were "enthusiastic" about hysterectomy, while the other's were "skeptical of its value." The residents in communities with wide disparities between surgical rates
still seemed to perceive themselves as having an equal level of
health and well-being. In addition, those with the less aggressive
surgeons did not seek their operations elsewhere.

Additional interesting and disturbing trends were provided by
Dicker and his associates in the *Journal of the American Medical Association* in 1982. Hysterectomy, it seemed, was a much more likely
scenario for you if you were black, or from the South. Even as the
overall numbers of operations declined from the late 1970s into
the 1980s, Southern women continued to undergo the most hysterectomies *and* at the youngest age. (The rate in the Northeast is the
lowest in the nation.)

Interestingly, if surgeons knew that they were being monitored,
it had a profound effect on how frequently they performed this

procedure. In 1972, in Saskatchewan, Canada, the health department noted a 72 percent increase in numbers of hysterectomies between 1964 and 1971. Growing concerned, they appointed a committee to perform surveillance on the overall numbers and underlying diagnoses of hysterectomies. They compiled a list of indications for hysterectomy and then analyzed all of the procedures in terms of whether they were indicated or not, based on their criteria. What they found was that, in the seven hospitals they examined, over a four-year period "the average proportion of unjustified hysterectomies had dropped from 23.7 percent at the time of the first review to 7.8 percent. . . . The total number of hysterectomies in the province dropped by 32.8 percent . . ." The authors were encouraged by their results, but expressed regret that such a committee had ever been necessary.

Last, but certainly not least, we discover some fascinating facts concerning hysterectomies and physicians themselves. For instance, when doctors' wives were studied, they were found to have an even *higher* rate of hysterectomy than the general female population. This might lead us to believe, therefore, that physicians truly had confidence in what they were doing, and were not performing unnecessary surgery for ulterior motives, such as monetary rewards. However, female gynecologists had much lower hysterectomy rates and seemed to perform about half as many of these procedures as did their male counterparts. Thus, if your doctor was a woman, you were statistically more likely to be spared a hysterectomy.

No researcher could definitively state whether the discrepancies repeatedly found from country to country and across various regions of the United States meant too much surgery in one place or too little surgery in another. To attempt to answer this controversy, at least where hysterectomy was concerned, doctors began to analyze the risks and benefits, the morbidity and mortality rates, and to come up with guidelines or indications for hysterectomy.

To understand this, first we have to take a look at why hysterectomies were (and still are) being done. Contrary to what most people might believe, cancer is the underlying reason for uterine removal only 10 percent of the time. Fibroids account for a significant portion of all hysterectomies: about 30 percent. Another 20 percent are performed to correct a relaxation of the pelvic structures which has allowed the uterus to prolapse. Endometriosis (when the uterine lining implants on structures outside of the uterus) is the diagnosis in another 15 percent of cases. (Endometriosis is the only diagnosis for which the numbers of hysterectomies are skyrocketing—by 176 percent—instead of falling.) A small number of hysterectomies (approximately 20 percent) seem to be performed for a variety of very rare conditions, such as obstetrical emergencies and severe infections (see Table 1.1).

However, of greatest concern and controversy are those hysterectomies which are performed for so-called cancer prevention and sterilization. According to Naomi Miller Stokes, in *The Castrated Woman*, 27 percent of all American women are unable to have children, largely because of hysterectomy. From Ann Arbor, Michigan, where 68.5 percent of all vaginal hysterectomies were performed for "socioeconomic" and "multiparity" reasons to Los Angeles where elective hysterectomy rates for sterilization rose in one hospital by 742 percent in two years, the overall rate of sterilization by hysterectomy increased by 293 percent between 1968 and 1970! This was particularly troubling because bilateral tubal ligation, a much simpler and safer procedure accomplishing sterilization, was common knowledge.

Perhaps the reason for the switch from minor surgery (tubal ligation) to major surgery (hysterectomy) can be explained by a fad of so-called prophylactic or preventative hysterectomies. In the early 1970s, one gynecologist, who out of compassion for his reputation, shall remain anonymous, declared to his colleagues that the time had come for their ranks to "recognize and recommend prophylactic elective total hysterectomy and bilateral salpingo-oophorectomy [removal of both fallopian tubes and ovaries] . . . as proper preventative medicine in obstetrics and gynecology." (One wonders what he would have thought of a urologist who might

Table 1.1   Hysterectomies performed in the United States: 1965–84

Diagnosis	Number
Fibroids	3,112,000
Prolapse	2,375,000
Endometriosis	1,586,000
Cancer	1,220,000
Miscellaneous conditions	2,933,000
Total	11,226,000

have recommended to him that his penis and testicles be amputated as "proper preventative medicine.") Be that as it may, this was not an extreme opinion of an eccentric gynecologist. The American College of Obstetrics and Gynecologists debated the controversy of elective hysterectomy at a meeting in 1971. In the end, supporters of the procedure significantly outclapped opponents, as measured on an audiometer. Dr. James H. Sammons, executive vice president of the American Medical Association sided with the majority. In 1977, he concurred that elective hysterectomies as a "convenient form of sterilization and . . . their prophylactic use to eliminate the possibility of uterine cancer in future years" was legitimate. While it might not be necessary in either case, he argued that it was "beneficial to women with excessive anxiety." Fortunately, as we shall soon see, society did not agree that hysterectomy was such a bargain. Feminists, congressional representatives, and insurance companies, among others, began to erode these ideas.

They were alarmed that of the half-million women having hysterectomies each year, approximately 2,000 would die, another 200,000 would suffer nonfatal complications, and over 100,000 would require blood transfusions. This was exclusive of the millions of health-care dollars expended on potentially unnecessary hysterectomies, not to mention time lost from employment or childcare duties.

There were shocking revelations of surgical abuse from all corners of society. For example, in a 1976 audit, Blue Cross/Blue Shield discovered that as many as 40 percent of hysterectomies performed in certain parts of the country resulted in the removal of totally normal organs for cancer or pregnancy prevention. As a result, during the mid to late 1970s, insurance companies began to require patients to obtain a second opinion before undergoing major surgery.

Congress launched an investigation of this matter in 1977 and reported in "Cost and Quality of Health Care" that hysterectomy was "questionable in 40 percent of cases including when it was done for obsessive fear of pregnancy and acute cancerphobia." The media had a field day reporting on unnecessary operations, and quoting doctors who candidly admitted that out came "a uterus or two each month to pay the rent." Of course, where doctors are concerned, lawyers are soon to follow. David Louisell and Harold Williams on the subject of medical malpractice wrote that, "Foremost among . . . surgical operations [performed without reasonable indications] are various gynecologic procedures."

If sterilization and cancer prevention did not justify hysterectomy, then what did? What were the valid "medical indications" for removal of the uterus? The response to this question came from many circles, primarily physicians and quality assurance committees.

Writing in a 1976 issue of the prestigious *New England Journal of Medicine*, gynecologist Valentina Clark Donahue declared the following to be "the appropriate indications for hysterectomy . . . .":

- Pre-malignant states and localized invasive cancers of the cervix, endometrium, ovaries or fallopian tubes;

- Symptomatic nonmalignant conditions of the uterus [such as fibroids] compressing adjacent pelvic structures and giving rise to repeated uterine bleeding not responsive to curettage [D&C];

- Uterine bleeding not responsive to hormonal therapy or uterine pain or bleeding in women in whom hormonal therapy is contraindicated, such as in women with adenomyosis [a condition whereby the lining of the endometrium grows inward, invading the muscle lining of the uterus];

- Diseases of the tubes and ovaries in which the uterus is not primarily involved but removed as part of the extirpation of these diseased adnexal appendages [pelvic organs] (for instance, chronic advanced tubal infections or severe endometriosis with extensive scarring of genital structures);

- Symptomatic descent or prolapse of the uterus due to disease or derangement of supporting structures;

- Removal of the uterus necessitated by operations for primary neoplasia [cancer] of adjacent structures;

- Obstetric catastrophes, including uncontrollable bleeding or uterine rupture;

- Therapeutic abortion in the first trimester [three months] of gestation [pregnancy] in selected cases for multiparous women [women with more than one child] who desire sterilization and for whom other forms of fertility control are contraindicated or not desired;

- Septic abortion [abortion resulting in uterine infection] not responsive to curettage [D&C] and medical therapy.

A year later, the American College of Obstericians and Gynecologists issued a policy statement that ranked gynecological surgery in order of necessity. So-called emergency situations would include hemorrhage of a tubal pregnancy, for example. Next in line were "mandatory" operations for "the presence of a malignancy." This was followed by "urgent" situations including "abnormal uterine bleeding which requires further diagnostic evaluation or definitive treatment." Then there were conditions for which surgery is "advisable," such as prolapse, and finally "elective" procedures for "family planning purposes."

The Professional Standards and Review Organization (PSRO), a hospital watchdog group responsible for auditing hospital stays and monitoring quality of care, basically agreed with only four of the above "medically appropriate indications for hysterectomy." They included: cancer and premalignant diseases, fibroids, abnormal bleeding conditions, and prolapsed uterus.

I believe that many of the above are poor reasons for hysterectomy, and represent a skewed and out-dated mentality now that alternative modes of treatment exist. In the following chapters, I hope to give you insight into why I am of this opinion. Yet, you can open any textbook today and you will still see some variation of these "medical indications" for hysterectomy.

The next logical question is, what if your hysterectomy was "indicated"? Did that mean you would be happier for it; would benefit from it; that it would improve the quality of your existence? Was it worth risking your life? Could the health-care-system budget tolerate surgery done for mere comfort and convenience? The jury is still out on these questions, despite numerous studies to attempt to answer them.

A researcher named Sonia Sandberg and her colleagues analyzed elective hysterectomies. Basically, they found that if a woman having her uterus removed for a benign process is destined to go on to develop cancer (a very small minority), then her life expectancy will increase by anywhere from roughly six to eight years. However, for the majority who do not develop cancer, but who would then be at increased risk of heart disease from having either a decline or cessation of ovarian function, there would be a decreased life expectancy. And, obviously for those unfortunate women who die from the surgery, over 39 years of life would be stolen from them.

Overall, Sandberg and her colleagues were of the opinion that elective hysterectomy *did* increase the quality of one's life. However, because it couldn't be predicted how women would perceive their inability to bear children (to some it would be an advantage; to others a disadvantage) or what psychological impact the removal of the uterus would have, these very significant factors were omitted from the study. In my opinion, these omissions are significant, and may have altered the authors' interpretation of the data concerning quality of life.

Harvard physician and epidemiologist Dr. Philip Cole studied the same question. He also found that a 35-year-old woman having an elective hysterectomy would benefit from an increased life expectancy, relief of some symptoms such as irregular uterine bleeding and economic gains. However, for 98.7 percent of the female population, no uterine cancer would be contracted and therefore there would be no increase in their life expectancy. *The overall 0.2 year increase in life expectancy (which was a statistical average), was exactly the same as the amount of time the average woman spends recovering from a hysterectomy!* Furthermore, each year of life saved in the name of cancer prevention would be costly and the years gained would be lived during old age—probably after age 75. Finally, the economic gains to society from the elimination of Pap smears, obstetrical care, D&Cs, contraceptives, and so forth for the women undergoing hysterectomy would be exceeded by its costs to the tune of $1.5 billion! In conclusion, said Dr. Cole, "Cancer prophylaxis cannot justify elective hysterectomy . . . the gains are uncertain but small and the potential health losses are great. We cannot assess the value of hysterectomy for contraception or other quality-of-life reasons, such as to reduce fear of cancer or to eliminate frequent, unpredictable bleeding."

Everyone agrees that hysterectomy can lead to complications, the specifics of which we will leave to a later chapter. However, the cruel irony in all of this is that, after numerous studies, meetings, and position papers, doctors remain embroiled in a bitter controversy regarding indicated versus necessary hysterectomies. This controversy strikes at the very livelihood of the obstetrician-gynecologist—his reason for existence. Because of this, old habits die hard, and no two doctors will give you exactly the same answer on this issue.

My opinion is that just because a condition may be a legitimate "indication" for surgery doesn't really mean that that condition *necessitates* surgery. For example, suppose a 40-year-old woman has a large fibroid, but she is unaware of its presence. It causes her absolutely no pain or excessive bleeding. Why then subject this woman to the perils and discomforts of a hysterectomy? The unfortunate fact is that the average woman attended by the average gynecologist will be "sold" a hysterectomy. She will be subtly convinced that her enlarging uterus might be an ominous precursor to cancer. With hysterectomy, the doctor will argue, not only will she be spared from this potential cancer, but from her monthly menstrual inconvenience and any unwanted pregnancies. After all, hadn't Dr. Wright said, in 1969, that after the last planned pregnancy the uterus becomes a "useless, bleeding, symptom-producing, potentially cancer-bearing organ" that should be removed?

The truth is that doctors don't advocate hysterectomy for women because they are a bad lot. They do so because it is "their operation." When I was in medical school, the gynecology residents in training were so eager to do surgery, we literally had a sign posted in the gynecology exam room that read, "Donate your uterus." Hysterectomy was our universal solution to nearly any problem. Remember that doctors like to find solutions to problems because their patients demand solutions and because they truly derive satisfaction from helping people. And a typically American solution to a problem is not to fix it, but to throw it out—or maybe replace it with something newer and better, such as artificial hormones.

Today, hysterectomy is dying hard because younger doctors are still being trained by older, traditional-minded physicians. New equipment is expensive, and difficult to master. Individual gynecologists don't appreciate the tremendous morbidity and mortality hundreds of thousands of procedures a year add up to. Nor do conventional doctors think about the immediate impact to a woman in terms of her six or eight weeks of incapacitation and what that means to her in lost income and neglected family responsibilities. From the surgeon's perspective, a "pelvic housecleaning" is very neat and tidy. They don't have to concern themselves with following a patient for future gynecologic problems. From the woman's perspective, she is entering a new era in her life, and she may not be prepared to cope with the loss she may experience in terms of her self-image as a complete woman. If there is any criticism that I have of the medical profession up to now, it is that we have *treated the uterus rather than treating the patient.*

That's the bad news. The good news is that this is changing. The vehicle for change has come from consumers of medical services demanding change and from technology being developed every day to respond to that demand. And the medical community is slowly but surely embracing this trend. Consider this passage from a letter by Dr. Stumpf in a recent issue of the *Journal of the American Medical Association.* He wrote of the future of in vitro fertilization—in other words, pregnancies conceived in a "test tube" then transferred to the mother's womb:

> Successful pregnancies, in both monkey and human subjects without ovaries have been reported as a result of ovum transfer and simple hormonal replacement. This information suggests that the uterus may no longer be considered a useless organ in all women following oophorectomy, since subsequent pregnancy is now clearly a realistic technical possibility. For this reason, is [sic] seems appropriate to reexamine the advisability of the traditional incidental excision of an otherwise healthy uterus at surgery to remove the ovaries in young women who may nevertheless desire later childbearing. The proposed benefits of incidental hysterectomy at the time of oophorectomy involve primarily a prophylaxis against later cancer in that organ. But endometrial cancer is usually detected easily, with low mortality after treatment, and cervical cancer may be effectively screened by conscientious use of [Pap] smears. The actual benefit of this prophylaxis may be questionable when balanced against the loss of childbearing potential. For comparison, there would certainly be no support for prophylactic removal of an otherwise healthy breast, although malignant neoplasms [cancer] in the breast are more common, more sinister, and more difficult to detect than cancers of the uterus.

Through advances in medical science there is now an alternative to nearly every indication for hysterectomy. A prolapse may safely be left alone, unless it is really bothersome. In that case, reconstructive surgery can be performed to repair rather than remove the offending structures. Laser surgery offers hope for the woman with endometriosis or fibroids, for which there is also myomectomy (the surgical excision of uterine fibroids). Abnormal bleeding may be treated by laser surgery or significantly reduced with hormonal therapy. Even certain precancerous lesions, depending on their location and the extent to which they have invaded the uterus, no longer mean automatic hysterectomy. The bottom line is that indicated hysterectomy does not equal necessary hysterectomy, as the following chapters will illustrate.

2

How Things Normally Work

Woman, in the interest of the race, is dowered with a set of organs peculiar to herself, whose complexity, delicacy, sympathies, and force are among the marvels of creation. If properly nurtured and cared for, they are a source of strength and power to her. If neglected and mismanaged, they retaliate upon their possessor with weakness and disease, as well of mind as of body.

—Edward H. Clarke, M.D., 1873.

From the beginning, the fertilized embryo is female. It is only in the presence of the male sex hormone, testosterone, that the genital ridge near the fetal tail will differentiate into a male. The male is formed out of the female by an elongation of the embryonic clitoris into a penis. By the time the fetus is a mere eight weeks old, she will have microscopic sex organs. The uterus and ovaries will be fully formed by six months. If she's fortunate, they will remain in a healthy, problem-free state throughout her life. These organs play a key role in the homeostasis of a woman which goes above and beyond the childbearing aspects. It is therefore essential to understand the normal functioning of the female reproductive tract before going any further in our discussion on hysterectomy.

A normal newborn baby girl will have a clitoris and vagina, cervix and uterus, as well as two fallopian tubes and ovaries. Her ovaries will already contain an excess of 400,000 ova, or eggs—the only ones she will ever produce in her lifetime. Unlike her male counterpart who will continuously manufacture millions of sperm until he is well into his later years, she will synthesize no more. But, once a month after puberty, she will release a single egg at ovulation.

If sperm are present, this union of one sperm with the egg will result in the formation of a fertilized embryo, and the cycle will begin again for the next generation.

Every month, a woman undergoes a series of events brought about by a complex interaction between the nervous, endocrine and reproductive systems of her body in preparation for a pregnancy. This is called the menstrual cycle.

The Menstrual Cycle and a Woman's Changing Hormones

Day one of the menstrual cycle is marked by the first day of menstrual flow. Depending on the woman, bleeding may commence anywhere from every 20 to 36 days, and last from two to eight days. During this time, she will shed only about two to three tablespoons of blood, but it will be mixed with equal amounts of other secretions from the cervix, endometrium, and vagina. This bleeding is triggered by signals ultimately originating in the brain.

Deep within the mid-brain, there is an area called the *hypothalamus*, which is responsible for a variety of functions in the human, including telling us when we are hungry, thirsty, sleepy, hot, or cold. The hypothalamus is an endocrine gland. This means that it secretes hormones, which are chemical substances synthesized in one place, and then transported through the bloodstream to exert an effect on a distant organ of the body. Specifically, the hypothalamus secretes hormones called *gonadotrophin releasing hormones* (GnRH) which are then sent via a specially designed circulatory system to another area of the brain, no larger than a pea, called the pituitary gland. The pituitary gland is divided into two sections. One section secretes hormones responsible for the uterine contractions that facilitate labor and delivery as well as the let-down of milk in the breastfeeding mother. The other section produces a host of chemicals regulating our growth and metabolism. It is also this portion of the gland that is stimulated by the hypothalamus to release its other major hormones, *luteinizing hormone* (LH) and *follicle stimulating hormone* (FSH) via the GnRH specific to each: LHRH and FSHRH, respectively. These then travel down to the ovary and trigger yet another round of activities, including the release of chemical substances here. The hormones produced in the ovary include: *estrogens, progesterone* (called progestin in vivo), and a small amount of male sex hormones called *androgens—* principally *testosterone.* The ovary itself is composed of hundreds of thousands of clusters of cells containing immature eggs. These units are called follicles.

At the start of the menstrual cycle, estrogen and progesterone levels are at their lowest. Low levels of these hormones exert what is known as a *feedback* effect on the hypothalamus, meaning that these depleted stores of estrogen and progesterone send a chemical message to the brain triggering the hypothalamus to release GnRH. The GnRH acts on the pituitary which then releases large amounts of FSH with a small quantity of LH. The follicle stimulating hormone then reaches the ovary where, as the name implies, it stimulates about a score of the immature follicles to mature. As they do, the follicles produce estrogens which act on the lining of the uterus, called the *endometrium.* The endometrium thickens, thus producing a rich carpet of nutrients in preparation for the implantation of a fertilized egg. It will be the lining of the uterus, specifically the placenta, that supports a developing fetus should pregnancy occur. Because of this growth and thickening of the endometrium during this time, this phase of the menstrual cycle, roughly days 6 through 13, is called the *proliferative phase.*

FSH and LH levels continue to mount until one follicle breaks away from the pack and continues its development while the others simply wither. Within this follicle, the egg is undergoing a process whereby the genetic material is being packaged into 23 separate chromosomes. These chromosomes will ultimately unite with 23 others provided by the male to produce the complete complement needed for a human being. The follicle increases its size five times over, and migrates to the surface of the ovary where it will eventually burst. When it ruptures, this follicle releases its egg in the process called *ovulation.* (Theoretically, this occurs on day 14.)

The egg floats away from the ovary and is captured by the fingerlike projections on the end of the fallopian tube. Once within the tube, it will take approximately three to four days for the ovum to travel to the uterus. Swept along on its journey by tiny hairlike structures called *cilia,* it is here in the fallopian tube that fertilization can take place. The ovum continues along the tube until it reaches the uterus where it takes another three days to implant in the lining if fertilized, or pass out of the body unnoticed if not. (If, for reasons that are not understood, the egg implants in the fallopian tube instead of in the uterus, an ectopic pregnancy occurs. This is a potentially life-threatening situation if not detected early on, because, as the embryo grows, it will stretch the tube beyond its limits until it eventually ruptures. This can cause the woman to bleed to death.)

Meanwhile, after the release of the egg, the ruptured follicle transforms itself into a specialized endocrine gland called the *corpus luteum* or "yellow body," so named because the presence of cholesterol gives it this characteristic color. Rising levels of luteinizing hormone assures this transformation and causes the newly-formed corpus luteum to produce estrogen and progesterone. This will maintain a pregnancy, should it occur, until the fetus is able to secrete its own hormones at about the eleventh week of pregnancy. Progesterone is the chemical that directs the endometrium to secrete nutrients for the developing fetus. Thus this phase is called the *secretory (luteal) phase.* It lasts from about day 15 to day 28 in the cycle.

If an embryo is in the uterus, it will produce yet another hormone known as *human chorionic gonadotrophin* (HCG). Chemically identical to LH, it takes over the role of the corpus luteum in stimulating estrogen and progesterone production. Pregnancy tests work on the principle of detecting rising levels of HCG as they are only present in pregnant women.

If no pregnancy has occurred, FSH and LH levels drop, the corpus luteum breaks down, and it no longer secretes progesterone and estrogens. Without the support of these hormones, particularly progesterone, the uterine lining degenerates. Blood vessels shrink and rupture, depriving the tissue of needed nutrient support. A combination of blood and tissue now passes out of the uterus through its opening in the cervix in the process called *menstruation.* Low levels of estrogen and progesterone then feed back to the hypothalamus beginning the process all over again. (See Figure 2.1.)

The average woman will go through approximately 500 menstrual cycles in her life from menarche (the onset of menstruation) to menopause (the end of menstrual cycles). Before puberty, there is no gonadotrophic activity in either the hypothalamus or

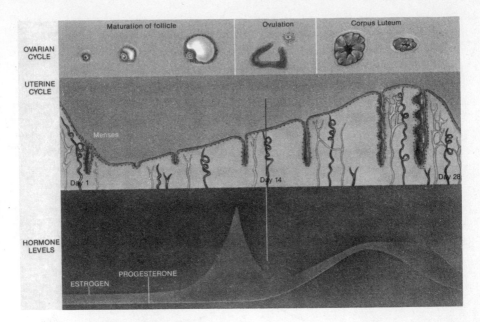

Figure 2.1   The menstrual cycle

the pituitary and thus there is no ovarian activity. For reasons not clearly understood, estrogens keep the pituitary in check until about the age of eight. Thereafter, the pituitary begins to secrete increasing amounts of gonadotrophic hormones which eventually lead up to the onset of menstrual periods.

Puberty and a Woman's Changing Anatomy

During puberty, the transition into adulthood, the female reproductive organs mature and prepare themselves for their adult functions, including procreation, pregnancy, and breastfeeding.

The female reproductive system is both internal and external. (See Figures 2.2, 2.3, and 2.4). Externally, of course, there are the breasts, vagina, and clitoris. At puberty, under the influence of increasing amounts of estrogens, the vagina enlarges, and fat becomes deposited in the *mons pubis* and *labia majora*. Likewise, the *labia minora* and clitoris enlarge. Pubic hair begins to grow on the perineum. (Hair development seems to come from the influences

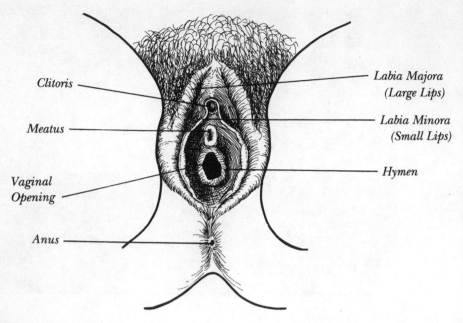

Clitoris

Meatus

Vaginal
Opening

Anus

Labia Majora
(Large Lips)

Labia Minora
(Small Lips)

Hymen

Figure 2.2   External female anatomy

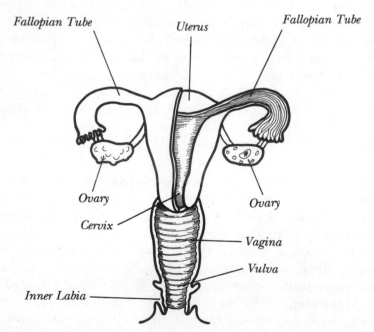

Fallopian Tube

Uterus

Fallopian Tube

Ovary

Cervix

Ovary

Vagina

Vulva

Inner Labia

Figure 2.3   Internal female anatomy, front view

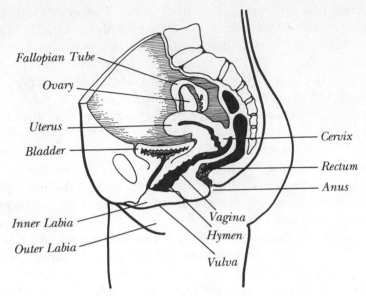

Figure 2.4   Internal female anatomy, side view

of the male sex hormones, the androgens, rather than from estrogen.) Within the vagina, the cellular structures are changing as well. The cells that line the walls of the vagina, called the "epithelium" change to a type that seems to be more resistant to trauma and infection.

The breasts also develop under the influences of estrogen. They grow larger, the nipples darken, and they initiate the development of the internal system of ducts and glands that will eventually produce milk for the newborn baby. However, the crucial completion of the milk-producing structures are under the influence of progesterone and prolactin. These hormones are produced by the ovary, placenta, and pituitary, respectively. In other words, while estrogens secreted during puberty lend the breasts their characteristically mature outward appearance, it is progesterone that is responsible for converting them to functioning organs.

If we imagine that we could look internally from a vantage point inside the vagina, the first thing that we would notice is a circular structure with an opening in the center. This is called the *cervix*, the "front door" to the uterus. In a woman who has never had children, the opening in the cervix, called the *os* is small and round. If a woman has had children, it is more elongated, and may have an irregular shape from birth trauma. The cervix contains nerves and blood vessels which may play a role in female sexual response. Likewise, it produces a natural lubricant to increase comfort and pleasure during intercourse, to facilitate the passage of sperm into the uterus, and to provide a hostile environment for bacterial foreign invaders. The cervix comprises the lower third of the *uterus*, the three-layered muscular organ that houses the developing fetus.

Shaped like an upside-down pear, the uterus enlarges two- to threefold during puberty to about the size of a fist. Inside the uterus, estrogen-mediated changes are occurring in the lining. It is thickening and developing more glandular tissue. The uterus of an adult woman consists of an outer layer of connective tissue and smooth muscle known as the *myometrium* and an inner, softer, more vascular endometrium which is sloughed every 28 days. Deeper than the endometrium is the *uterine cavity* which is no larger than a slit in the nonpregnant female, but it is capable of expanding to accommodate a seven- or eight-pound baby.

Scientists are still making discoveries about the functions of the uterus independent of supporting a fetus. It is known to produce two vital groups of chemicals. The first of these are *beta endorphins*, the body's natural painkillers, which produce a mild euphoria and sense of well-being. The second group, the *prostaglandins*, serve a variety of functions. Because they cause contraction of smooth muscle, it is the prostaglandins that are to blame for menstrual cramping. They are also believed to be protective against heart disease because of their role in preventing blood clotting.

Branching out from the fundus, or top of the uterus, on either side are the fallopian tubes. Four inches long, they attach to the uterus via a nearly microscopic opening, and then end, just short of the ovaries, with fringelike projections called *fimbriae*. As mentioned earlier, the fallopian tube, also called the *oviduct* (or egg tube) is the vestibule between the ovary and uterus where sperm unites with egg. Fallopian tubes in the mature female have more glandular tissue. In addition, following puberty, they contain greater numbers of increasingly active cilia which are constantly beating in the direction of the uterus. This obviously aids the ovum in its monthly journey.

Perhaps the most critical and complex of the female reproductive organs are the ovaries. Almond-shaped and weighing about a quarter of an ounce each, they rest in the pelvic cavity adjacent to the fallopian tubes. To review, the ovaries contain thousands of egg-bearing follicles—the sites of estrogen, progesterone, and androgen production. They synthesize these steroid hormones using cholesterol as a building block. It is theorized that active ovarian function therefore prevents buildup of cholesterol in the arteries of the body and thus protects women from cardiovascular disease until menopause.

In addition to progesterone, women synthesize three types of estrogens: *estradiol, estrone,* and *estriol,* as well as two different male sex hormones. (All of these chemicals are present in men as well, but obviously in differing proportions. It is believed that the sex drive in the female is related to her level of the male hormone, testosterone.) Estrogens, progesterone, and androgens are also made, to a lesser extent, within the adrenal glands. These are small organs attached to the kidneys. Some very recent studies seem to indicate that women continue to produce estrogens and androgens even after menopause, both in the adrenals and ovaries, and that they may play a role in regulating blood pressure in addition to their already established functions.

Aside from the reproductive organs, increased output of estrogen from the ovary during puberty causes changes in the adolescent's overall physical appearance. Her skin is softer and her body more curvaceous from selective fat deposition. She experiences the characteristic adolescent growth spurt as well as a molding of her pelvis into the broad, oval structure necessary for childbirth. Throughout her premenopausal life, estrogen will also stimulate new bone growth, safeguarding her against the ravages of osteoporosis.

Menopause and a Woman's Changing Physiology

Medically defined, menopause is said to have occurred if a woman has had absolutely no monthly bleeding for a period of at least one year. Interestingly, for most of human existence, women statistically did not live long enough to experience menopause. They generally died from infectious diseases or childbirth years before any decline in ovarian function. Therefore, the collective experience of women facing the changes inherent in menopause is very recent history, and much of it is still misunderstood. In stark contrast to our great grandmothers who lived a mere century ago, women in their menopausal years are not waiting out their final years. They are active in society, often engaged in first or second careers after having raised a family.

There are three distinct stages to menopause. The first is the premenopause, which is a time when there is a steady decline in ovarian function. In much the same way as they begin in the teenaged years, the menstrual periods are irregular and sometimes occur without actual ovulation. Before the onset of menopause, a woman may experience heavier periods, lighter periods, and/or erratic changes in the pattern of her cycle. As mentioned before, once she has had no periods for one year, a woman is considered to have undergone menopause. This means that she has no active follicles remaining in her ovary. She can no longer conceive or menstruate. However, her ovary does continue to synthesize hormones in small amounts and this is key to the other roles they play in her body, mainly related to heart and bone health.

Most women experience menopause in their late 40s or early 50s. Like menarche, the actual age varies between individual women and may similarly be related to such factors as race, heredity, nutrition, and general health.

The final stage is the postmenopause when ovarian mass decreases by 50 percent and ovarian hormone production wanes.

There are several distinct physiologic changes that a decline in estrogen production causes in women. The obvious one is the absence of menstrual periods. Two notable others are: hot flashes and drying of the vaginal walls with a loss of their previous elasticity. While it is not completely understood, estrogen seems to stabilize the blood vessels, preventing them from enlarging and shrinking in an irregular manner. When estrogen is no longer readily available, there is unpredictable dilation and constriction, which causes the sometimes sudden and intense sweating and chills that women experience.

In addition, just as they had developed during puberty, now, the breasts, pelvic organs, and vaginal area shrink as fat and glandular tissue thin out. Thinning vaginal tissue becomes more easily irritated. This may lead to painful intercourse or an inflammation of the vagina sometimes called *atrophic vaginitis*. Estrogen, protective of the heart and skeleton, is no longer present to counteract the effects of arteriosclerosis and weakened bones.

Finally, women may encounter a host of psychological symptoms ranging from moodiness and fatigue to depression. Researchers are at work studying how much of this is physiologic and how much is environmental or emotional, related to such life events as children leaving home, spouses dying, disease becoming more prevalent, and so forth.

How these changes may best be dealt with will be discussed in Chapter Eight. For now, we move on to the disease entities, signs and symptoms women may experience when something goes awry in this intricate system of female anatomy and physiology.

Part 2

The Alternatives

Yesterday morning I arrived at the hospital to find that the woman whose hysterectomy I watched last week was going back to the operating room for the third time. Last week they took her back to remove a blood clot from the site of surgery, and yesterday they opened her and cleaned out all the clotted blood and pus, which should probably have been removed the first time they took her back. . . .

I found myself staring at the tubes coming out of the woman's belly and vagina, wondering if the women would be so willing to have surgery if they knew what was being done to them. No one should be asleep for surgery.

—Michelle Harrison, M.D.
A Woman In Residence

Fibroid Tumors of the Uterus

The existence of this function [menstruation] alone, makes it impossible for women—except in peculiar individual cases—to pursue the same avocations and follow the same mode of life as man.

—Dr. Frederick Hollick, 1840

In reality, fifteen or twenty days out of twenty-eight (we may say nearly always), woman is not only an invalid, but a wounded one. She ceaselessly suffers from love's eternal wound.

—Jules Michelet, 1868

What Are Fibroids?

Marlene had only just passed her thirty-fifth birthday when she first faced needing a hysterectomy. For several years her menstrual periods had become heavier and heavier to the point that she now needed to use two tampons and a pad simultaneously. Not only did she dread the embarrassment of a public accident, but wondered if she was at risk for toxic shock syndrome. She literally felt robbed of one week every month when she would be practically incapacitated. Marlene's gynecologist diagnosed multiple fibroids and recommended hysterectomy to put an end to her misery. But, although she was still single, Marlene hoped to have children someday. She began to explore the alternatives.

Fibroids are responsible for approximately 200,000 hysterectomies per year. The most common "benign" disease entities of the female reproductive tract, they are present in anywhere from 30 to 50 percent of all women between 40- and 50-years old, afflicting twice as many black women as white women. Women who have never had children and nonsmokers also seem to be at greater risk of developing fibroids, although no one really knows why. It has been noted that estrogen may somehow play a role in their growth and development, because fibroids are never seen before puberty, and seem to shrink after menopause. In addition, fibroids tend to worsen during pregnancy, when estrogen levels are high. Furthermore, in the early days of higher dose birth control pills, users seemed to be more predisposed to fibroids (again due to the influences of estrogen?). However, at least one recent study seems to indicate that this may no longer be the case.

The term fibroid refers to the fact that the tissue comprising a fibroid is fibrous-like. However, fibroids are actually smooth muscle in origin. That's why the more precise, but less commonly used medical term, *leiomyoma* is actually more appropriate (*leio* means smooth; *my* means muscle; and *oma* means tumor or growth).

No one really understands why or how fibroids develop, but they are believed to start out as one tiny smooth muscle cell that goes awry in the myometrium (middle layer of the uterus). From there, a myoma may remain within the myometrium or insinuate itself in the outer or innermost layers of the uterus. Fibroids within the central muscle layer of the uterus are called *intramural* or *interstitial* tumors. Those on the outside protruding into the abdominal cavity are so-called *subserous* or *serosal* types, and those that invade the endometrium, *submucous* leiomyomas. (See Figure 3.1.)

They can occasionally migrate out from the uterus, invading the cervix, surrounding ligaments or, rarely, other abdominal organs containing smooth muscle. (Fibroids have even been found in the stomach and intestine.) Like all living tissue, they require oxygen and nutrients transported to them via the bloodstream. When fibroids occasionally develop a blood supply outside of the uterus, they are termed *parasitic* fibroids. If they should elongate and grow a stalk (only in the case of the submucous and subserous types) they are called *pedunculated*.

Fibroids can be singular, but more commonly are multiple. They can be so tiny that they are visible only under a microscope, or so large as to weigh 30 pounds. Furthermore, a woman's symptoms may have no direct bearing on the number or size of the tumors. Indeed, she may have one the size of a full-term pregnancy that causes her little or no discomfort!

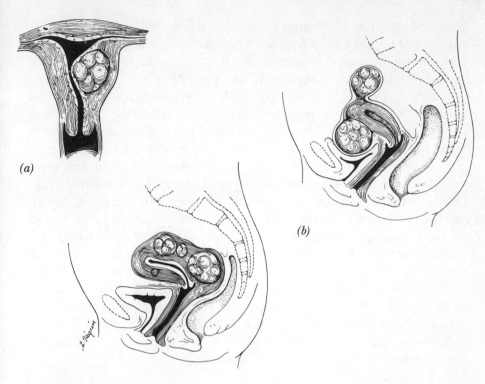

Figure 3.1   Uterine fibroids—Benign growths of muscle tissue named according to the location in the uterus: (a) submucous (inside the endometrium), (b) subserous (outside the uterine wall), and (c) intramural (within the uterine wall).

The Symptoms

Bleeding

Generally speaking, when a woman does have symptoms from her fibroids, those symptoms are heavier flow and perhaps more painful menstrual periods. She may suffer from a gushing flow or the passage of blood clots, and may experience some of the signs of the anemia that heavy bleeding can cause, such as pallor, fatigue, or dizziness. However, fibroids can also cause an abnormal *pattern* of bleeding, such as staining between periods or bleeding after menopause. This is less common, and any woman having this kind of bleeding should not automatically attribute it to fibroids (even if she is known to have them). Other potentially more serious causes of abnormal bleeding have to be ruled out. (For the record, one-half of 1 percent of fibroids become malignant. From a practical perspective, what that means is that, in my 25 years of gynecological practice, I have seen only two patients whose fibroids were cancerous. A cancerous fibroid, or leiomyosarcoma, is suspected when a fibroid is observed to enlarge at an unusually rapid rate.)

The severity of the bleeding associated with fibroids has a great deal to do with their location. For example, in contrast to subserous fibroids, which may cause few symptoms relative to their size, even a small intramural or submucous fibroid can cause hemorrhaging. This is because fibroids that extend through the thickness of the uterine wall and into the endometrium below have large blood vessels coursing through them. During menstruation, when the endometrium is sloughed, these vessels open up and literally pour out blood. Scores of patients suffering from these types of fibroids tell horrifying tales of being afraid to wear white dresses or even to go to work for fear of the opening of the floodgates during their periods. Ironically, as long as the blood supply to these fibroids remains so generous, these women may experience little or no *dysmenorrhea*—painful menstrual cramping.

Pain

As mentioned earlier, fibroids require blood to transport the nutrients necessary to maintain them. If, however, the blood vessels are too few or too narrow, as when a large fibroid is anchored by a small stalk, there may be inadequate support to keep it viable. It may then begin to degenerate. The death of the fibroid causes an inflammatory response as the body tries to rid itself of this dying tissue. Inflammation causes pain, usually in the form of cramping as the uterus contracts.

Depending on its location, a fibroid may cause different types of pain. A submucous fibroid, for instance, may cause laborlike pains as the uterus tries to expel it through the cervix during menstruation. Pedunculated fibroids can become twisted on their stalks causing sudden and intense pain as the blood supply is abruptly shut down. Intramural fibroids, like adenomyosis—a condition we will discuss in the next chapter—may cause a generally tender, achy uterus. Finally, fibroids located on the outside of the uterus may impinge on other pelvic structures, causing so-called pressure symptoms.

Pressure Symptoms

Many women with fibroids suffer from a sensation of pressure in the back, legs, or lower abdominal region. For example, if a fibroid rests on vessels supplying blood to the legs, a woman may develop varicose veins and pain with prolonged standing. Fibroids located on the back of the uterus may cause backaches or rectal symptoms, and with fibroids in the front of the uterus, a woman may experience painful intercourse, or have to urinate frequently. Bladder problems may abound with certain strategically located tumors—even causing conditions where the woman cannot adequately urinate. This retention of urine predisposes a woman to infections because stagnant urine is a perfect medium for bacterial growth. Eventually, the urine within the bladder overflows uncontrollably, resulting in incontinence.

Pregnancy-Related Problems

Fibroids may be responsible for problems related to pregnancy literally from start to finish. Infertility may result from the presence of a fibroid within the uterine lining causing interference with the implantation of the fertilized egg. However, this condition is most often reversed when the offending fibroid is removed. Indeed, many women with fibroids conceive without difficulty. This leads one to believe that, perhaps in those women who don't, another factor, such as blocked fallopian tubes or endometriosis may be the actual cause.

The pregnant woman with fibroids requires expert obstetrical care and careful monitoring. With small fibroids, the odds are on her side to have a safe, usually vaginal, delivery of a healthy baby. Larger fibroids may pose special challenges to the patient and her doctor. This is because uterine fibroids increase their size greatly during pregnancy when estrogen levels are high, and this may place the woman with fibroids more at risk for miscarriage, premature birth, or postpartum hemorrhage.

What a Pelvic Exam Can Tell You

Diagnosing fibroids usually begins with the pelvic exam. There is more to the annual check-up than a Pap smear. First, the external genitalia are examined for any signs of infectious or cancerous lesions. Then, the speculum is inserted to separate the walls of the vagina, thus allowing your doctor to view the cervix. Normally, the cervix is pink and round, with a tiny opening in its center. It is that opening that expands to 4 inches during childbirth to allow the passage of the newborn baby from the uterus. The cervix should be free of discharge, growths, and erosion. (Occasionally, there will appear to be a fleshy protrusion present which may be a small fibroid or polyp.)

After locating the cervix, your doctor then takes a small wooden stick, called a spatula, and scrapes off the superficial layer of cells from the surface. These, along with cells collected with a cotton swab from the cervical opening itself are sent to the laboratory for examination. The Pap test (named for its inventor, Dr. George Papanicolaou), classifies these cells into various types, which will be described in Chapter Six. At this point, other specimens may be collected—to check for infections, for example, if they are suspected.

Afterward, the speculum is removed, and the doctor performs a bimanual examination. This is so-named because it requires the placement of both hands—one inside the vagina and one on the lower abdomen—so that the uterus and ovaries may be palpated between them. An experienced practitioner can discover, by feeling the contours of these internal organs, whether they are normal in size and shape. It is during this portion of the pelvic exam that fibroids are generally discovered. Indeed, they may merely be a coincidental finding in a woman who is having no problems with her menses but who, on exam, is found to have an enlarged and irregularly shaped uterus.

Last, but not least, is the rectal exam. While many patients would prefer to omit this portion of the examination as they may find it distasteful or uncomfortable, it is absolutely essential. Especially in a woman whose uterus is angled slightly backward, the rectal exam permits the doctor to explore the underside of the uterus and to check for ovarian tumors. At the same time, a simple and quick test for rectal bleeding may be performed. This aids in the diagnosis of certain gastrointestinal conditions, including bowel cancer. It is important to emphasize here that *unless you have had a rectal exam, you have not had a complete pelvic exam.*

The Standard Response

A D&C is the "bread and butter" of gynecologic surgery. That's how it was described to me over the sinks one day as the attending surgeon and I were scrubbing to do the operation.
—Michelle Harrison, M.D.
From A Woman In Residence

"Just A 'Dusting and Cleaning'"

A "dusting and cleaning" is the patient's nickname for the ubiquitous D&C (dilation and curettage). Easily the most commonly performed gynecological procedure, literally millions of women undergo one every year. After anesthetizing the woman, the doctor first inserts instruments to gradually widen the cervical opening and then uses other surgical tools, passed through this opening, to scrape away the endometrium. The gynecologist may also obtain tissue samples that will be sent to the laboratory in an effort to diagnose the cause of the bleeding.

The D&C has traditionally been a very popular procedure because it has been believed to be both diagnostic and therapeutic for women with heavy menstrual periods or abnormal bleeding patterns. However, critics of the D&C, such as myself, believe that it's outdated and doesn't go far enough in helping women. To begin with, the traditional D&C is a blind procedure whereby the doctor doesn't directly view the uterine lining and thus must rely on what he feels with the curette to diagnose the presence of fibroids or other abnormal growths. In addition, because he can't see what he's doing, the gynecologist cannot be sure he has eradicated the problem or sampled the key portion of the endometrium for lab analysis. Furthermore, the D&C hardly ever goes far enough in curing the bleeding, depending on the underlying problem. Specifically, my research, as well as studies conducted by Dr. Frank Loffer, have shown that at least one-third of pathology is missed during curettage. Dr. Loffer's work also demonstrated that a D&C provides only temporary relief of bleeding because it only scrapes off the superficial layer of the uterine lining. The foundation of the lining remains, allowing for a recurrence. As a result, many women need repeated D&Cs. The "standard response" after three unsuccessful D&Cs is hysterectomy!

Myomectomy versus Hysterectomy

Myomectomy is a surgical procedure whereby the fibroid tumors are removed and the remainder of the uterus is preserved and reconstructed. (See Figure 3.2.) It has been performed for years when the gynecologist is told by his patient that she desires children. However, because this surgery is more complex and time-consuming, traditional physicians recommend hysterectomy, sometimes with oophorectomy, to women in their 40s as a more "appealing" and permanent solution to their fibroid problem. It is true that once the uterus is gone, the fibroids will have no opportunity to grow back and cause any troublesome pain and bleeding. It is also true that hysterectomy is a technically less difficult operation (though not to the doctor who is accustomed to performing myomectomy). Traditional physicians claim that myomectomy may cause greater blood loss thus increasing the chance of a transfusion. There is also a slightly higher death rate and, depending on the woman's age, always the chance that the fibroids will recur. However, with modern techniques this can be averted. Furthermore, a woman, regardless of her childbearing plans or potential, may have physical and emotional reasons for wanting to preserve her uterus and her feelings must be respected.

> *Claire was such a woman. At age 45, Claire came to me complaining of extremely heavy periods. Though in agony, she was emphatic about keeping her uterus. After removing nine fibroids from her uterus, I was taken to task by one of my colleagues who could not begin to understand why I had not talked her into a more "sensible" hysterectomy. Yet, after her surgery, Claire was left with an essentially normal-sized uterus, and was delighted when her next period was completely normal. Furthermore, she attained menopause without any recurrence of her symptoms.*

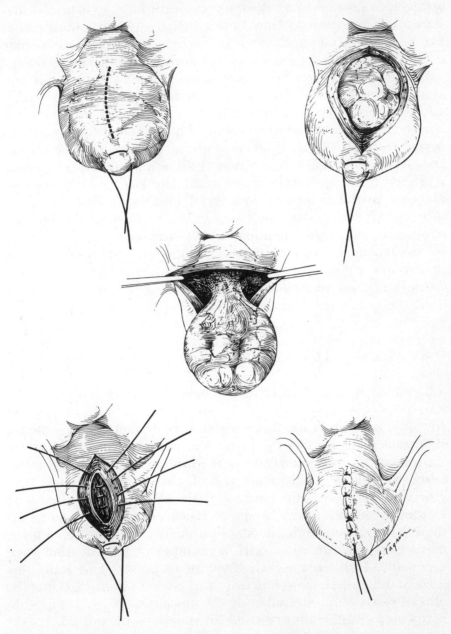

Figure 3.2   The myomectomy procedure—An incision is made in the uterus and the fibroid is excised, leaving the main body of the uterus intact.

Performed by a gynecologist experienced in reconstructive surgery, as myomectomy is sometimes now known, it is safe, and may allow a woman to "buy time" so that she can complete her family or reach menopause—a time when her fibroids will recede and her symptoms lessen. In my opinion, there is certainly no age at which a woman "needs" to have a hysterectomy; only conditions that may warrant one. However, a woman must be well-informed as to her alternatives and her odds for success with myomectomy. These are somewhat age-dependent. That is, if a woman is 30 with severe pain and bleeding, she may go for 10 years after a myomectomy before she again experiences difficulties. Now she's 40 and is still menstruating. But, in the interim, she has had 10 symptom-free years with her uterus. However, if a woman is 40, the chances are overwhelming that she's not going to have problems after myomectomy because menopause will intercede.

We'll come back to myomectomy later, but first let's take a look at how modern diagnostic and treatment techniques have broadened the "standard response" to the management of fibroids.

The Modern Approach to Diagnosis

Hysteroscopy: The End to the Blind D&C

In 1805, a German military physician of Italian descent named Philipp Bozzini became the first scientist to devise an instrument through which one could observe the hidden cavities of the human body. He called his invention the "Lichtleiter" and it was little more than a long, thin lantern made of tin and covered with leather. It utilized a wax candle as its source of illumination. Although it received a brief flurry of publicity, including an endorsement from the Archduke Karl, a member of the Austrian royal family, the Lichtleiter soon fell victim to politics and jealousies. Bozzini disappeared into obscurity and it wasn't until 1869 that the idea of examining internal body cavities was once again raised by Pantaleoni. Pantaleoni first used his narrow tube and a kerosene lamp to examine the cause of heavy bleeding in an elderly woman. Over the next century, scientists and physicians continued to perfect various scopes to examine the genitourinary tract, adding more complex lenses, cold light fiberoptics, and introducing fluids and suctioning devices into the uterus. These were used to minimize distortion from blood and debris, and to maximize visibility of the structures within the cavity.

Today, the descendent of the Lichtleiter is called the hysteroscope (see Figure 3.3). Hysteroscopy is a low-risk procedure during which the physician introduces a fiberoptic scope into the uterus, in the presence of either a sugar or saltlike fluid or carbon dioxide gas. These substances enlarge the uterine cavity making it easier to examine. The patient requires minimal sedation and feels little discomfort during the examination. Hysteroscopy can be performed in a doctor's office or in the hospital. Afterward, the woman goes home and can resume her normal activities in a few days. The side effects are generally very minor, and may include some mild cramping or light bleeding afterward. Very rarely (about once in every 10,000 patients) a woman may have an allergic reaction to the sugarlike fluid used.

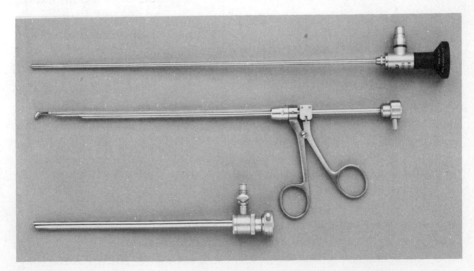

Figure 3.3 A hysteroscope—A fiberoptic scope inserted through the cervix to view the interior of the uterus.

The advantage over the D&C, of course, is that the doctor is able to evaluate the entire lining of the uterus, and can usually determine the cause of the woman's symptoms. The gynecologist can detect polyps, fibroids, suspicious tumors, and can sample the endometrium at the same time. Several studies have now confirmed what common sense seems to tell us: that hysteroscopy is more sensitive and more accurate than dilation and curettage. In 1985, two physicians, Dr. Goldrath and Dr. Sherman, found that "large numbers" of polyps and fibroids were missed on blind D&C because "less than half of the uterine cavity had been curetted in sixty percent of patients and less than a fourth of the cavity in sixteen percent"!

In 1987, I conducted a retrospective study of nearly 300 women evaluating the efficacy of D&C by hysteroscopy and found results similar to Dr. Goldrath and Dr. Sherman. Hysteroscopy was routinely performed prior to curettage. After identifying 185 patients with pathology such as polyps, we found that most patients still retained their polyps after curettage. Most required multiple attempts at removal. Only with hysteroscopy could we tell that the pathology had been completely removed. In addition, hysteroscopy spared other patients the need to return for repeated curettages while continuing to suffer from their symptoms because an examination of the entire uterus was able to be conducted at once.

One final advantage to this procedure is that instruments may also be introduced via the hysteroscope to treat abnormal bleeding conditions, making operative hysteroscopy a simpler, safer, and more convenient alternative to hysterectomy for millions of women.

Ultrasound: Something Old and Something New

Ultrasound (sonogram) utilizes the emission of intermittent high-frequency sound waves which bounce off the structures within the pelvic cavity in certain patterns depending on their densities. These patterns are then interpreted by a computer and conveyed on a television screen to depict the size, shape, and any irregularities to the uterus and ovaries. Ultrasound is a very safe, noninvasive diagnostic test during which a physician or technician applies a conducting jelly to the abdomen and then passes a metal object called a *transducer* over it to record the sound waves. No dyes or Xrays are involved. The test takes about 30 minutes to perform.

Traditionally, sonograms have been performed through the abdomen, and the only discomfort to be anticipated is that a full bladder is required so that a clear view of the pelvic organs may be obtained. Pitfalls to abdominal ultrasound, which may result in a less than optimal picture, include instances when a woman is overweight, or when there is scar tissue or intestinal gas present—all of which may obscure the picture. To overcome many of these obstacles, I use transvaginal ultrasound extensively in my practice.

During transvaginal ultrasound, a full bladder is unnecessary and that therefore eliminates this complaint by patients concerning the sonogram procedure. A plastic probe covered with a lubricant is inserted into the vagina, where it can then be positioned in different angles to directly view the uterus, ovaries, fallopian tubes, and the area behind the uterus known as the *cul-de-sac.*

Several studies support the notion that the transvaginal route permits a better quality image and provides more information to the doctor and the patient about the status of her pelvic structures. For example, in a recent issue of *Radiology,* Dr. Mendelson and her colleagues compared transabdominal and transvaginal ultrasound in 200 women. They discovered that transvaginal image quality was better overall in 79 to 87 percent of all scans. Specifically, because the vaginal probe is closer to the organs being studied, they got a clearer view of the uterus (including finer endometrial detail), the fallopian tubes (especially important when searching for an ectopic pregnancy), and the ovaries (except when they were in a high position). The image quality was unaffected by abdominal scarring, obesity, bowel, or the need for a full bladder. Because it is quicker and less uncomfortable for most patients, women tend to prefer this approach. It will probably be the way of the future for most gynecologic ultrasound.

However, on occasion, a fibroid may be mistaken on ultrasound for other abnormalities. Therefore, other imaging tests—more expensive and more accurate—including the CAT scan and the MRI, are occasionally performed to clarify the sonographic findings.

CATs and MRIs: The Alphabet Soup of Diagnostic Tests

"CAT" stands for computerized axial tomography; this is a specialized form of X ray in which the organ being studied is x-rayed in a series of very thin sections or slices. These are then analyzed by a computer that assimilates them into a more three-dimensional and detailed view than is possible by conventional X ray.

"MRI" or magnetic resonance imaging is the newest type of clinical imaging technique. Unlike the CAT scan, it does not use X rays. Instead, it relies on a powerful magnet which exerts a force on the subatomic particles (protons) in your body tissue. Like the CAT scan, it utilizes a computer to analyze the patterns the particles form as they return to their normal state after being energized by the magnet. The computer creates a detailed picture of the body structure being scanned which is even more complete than ultrasound or CAT scanning.

Today's Treatment Options

Today, we can offer the woman suffering from fibroids a variety of medical and surgical therapies to treat her condition—*all of which thankfully fall short of hysterectomy.* Which therapy she selects, in consultation with her gynecologist, is dependent on a variety of factors, including her age, symptoms, and childbearing plans. Let's examine the options.

Careful Observation

As we've already noted, if there were a way to look inside the uterus of every woman past age 40, chances are that more than half would have a myoma, and many of them would not be aware of it. This is important to realize because it points to the fact that we do not have to intervene in every case where fibroids are discovered. Careful observation of the progress of that fibroid may be all that is necessary, particularly in a woman who is having no symptoms or who is nearing menopause.

In my patients who fall into this category, I perform a baseline vaginal ultrasound, and then monitor them with pelvic exams every 6 to 12 months to follow their symptoms and any significant change in the growth of the fibroid. For example, if a woman has a fibroid that initially measured two centimeters (about three-quarters of an inch) and it doubles, it is still not bound to be problematic (providing she is having no symptoms). However, a four-centimeter myoma that doubles *is* now significant, and a decision should be made as to how to proceed. If, for instance, this woman is young, a fibroid that size might interfere with a planned pregnancy so treatment should be instituted to lessen the chance of complications. But if this woman is nearing menopause, she may elect to shrink the fibroid with medical therapy until the natural estrogen depletion associated with menopause takes over causing the fibroid to recede permanently.

Medical Therapy: The GnRH or LHRH Agonists

In Chapter Two, where we discussed normal female physiology, you will recall mention of chemicals produced within the brain, notably the hypothalamus and the pituitary, which then influence the production of estrogen in the ovary throughout the menstrual cycle. Among those chemicals produced by the hypothalmus are so-called gonadotrophin releasing hormone or luteinizing releasing hormone (GnRH and LHRH, respectively). It is now possible for women suffering from fibroids (and a variety of other estrogen-dependent conditions) to take synthetic versions of these hormones with the end result of shrinking their tumors.

Specifically, when a woman takes a GnRH agonist, usually via monthly, long-acting injections, she initially stimulates her pituitary gland to produce a follicle-stimulating hormone. This, in turn, causes the ovary to produce estrogen—as in the normal menstrual cycle. However, under the influence of these artificially introduced chemicals, eventually (usually after a period of two weeks), because of constant stimulation of the body's sensitive feedback controls, the pituitary becomes *downregulated*. This means that this bombardment of external chemicals mimicking GnRH has exhausted the pituitary's own gonadotrophins. The continued artificial hormone maintains that state. As a result, the ovary produces no estrogen and fibroids decrease to about half of their original size!

While this is a promising, nonsurgical approach to the treatment of fibroids, it has some significant drawbacks. The first is that GnRH agonists to date have no convenient route of administration. They do not retain effectiveness when taken by mouth or, for example, as a vaginal suppository. They have to be injected daily, or monthly using what is known as a long-acting "depot." This is a site underneath the skin where a long-acting version of the drug is implanted. They may also be administered intranasally; however, the nasal method was only recently approved by the Food and Drug Administration (FDA) and its long-term effectiveness has yet to be evaluated. A major drawback to its long-term use may be the irritation of the nasal membranes. In addition, this medication is extremely expensive.

Perhaps the greatest drawback to the GnRH treatment is its lack of permanence. In other words, as soon as treatment is stopped, many fibroids quickly grow back to their original size. One study followed women on GnRH agonists from the time they began therapy until from two to six months after they had discontinued the injections. While the fibroids had shrunk by anywhere from 62 to 100 percent of their original volume as long as the injections continued, once off the medication *40 percent* of these women's fibroids had returned to their pretreatment size, and, in some cases, had actually exceeded it! At the present time, physicians are fearful of keeping women on these drugs for the long term because of the potentially harmful effects of years of estrogen suppression, in terms of heart and bone disease.

Why, then, pursue this form of therapy? First, it may tide women over who are naturally approaching menopause and who may then avoid surgery all together. Second, it may be used in women who are unable to undergo surgery due to a variety of health complications until those complications can be overcome or stabilized. Last, but not least, short-term GnRH therapy may be administered to all women facing fibroid surgery to lessen its complexity—the medication shrinks the fibroids significantly, lessens the amount of bleeding, and eases the removal of the tumors. Recent studies show that the concomitant use of estrogen with GnRH relieves the anti-estrogen effect without allowing regrowth. This concept is new and is undergoing further study.

The Anti-Estrogens

Aside from the GnRH agonists, some doctors have employed medications called "anti-estrogens" and/or "antiprogesterones." Perhaps the most well-known of these is Danazol (Danocrine). Like the

GnRH agonists, they shrink myomas by blocking estrogen production. They, too, have been effective in reducing bleeding and pain in chronic sufferers. However, unlike GnRH, these chemicals are "androgens," meaning that they are analogs of the male sex hormone, testosterone. As a result, they seem to be less effective, and to cause more side effects to women than the former group. Many women are troubled by the particular side effects of male sex hormones, which may include: deepening of the voice, acne, and hair growth, particularly on the face.

Nonsteroidal Anti-Inflammatory Medications

For years, women have been taking a group of medications called "nonsteroidal anti-inflammatory drugs" to decrease the painful cramping associated with menstruation. Two of the most well-known drugs in this category are Ibuprofen(Motrin) and Naproxen(Naprosyn). They are believed to relieve pain by inhibiting the release of chemicals called prostaglandins that are responsible for the inflammation and uterine contractions known to occur during menstruation. However, patients and scientists have observed an interesting phenomenon that seems to accompany long-term use of these medications. Not only is the pain reduced, but so is the flow. In other words, women taking Motrin or Naprosyn notice after a while that their periods are shorter and lighter than before. Therefore, several gynecologists decided to investigate whether fibroid sufferers with symptoms of severe pain and bleeding would experience the same results. Unfortunately, their findings were disappointing. Women with myomas are unaffected by the use of nonsteroidal anti-inflammatory drugs, suggesting that other, as yet unknown, factors may play a role in their heavy bleeding and painful periods.

State-of-the-Art Laser Hysteroscopy

Women whose fibroids cause them intractable bleeding need no longer turn to hysterectomy as the only answer to their dilemma. Through the lens of the hysteroscope, a surgeon can now aim a laser and, like a space warrior in a battle out of science fiction, literally vaporize the offending tissue and blood vessels.

The term *laser* is an acronym for light amplification by stimulated emission of radiation. This technique takes an intense and sharply focused beam of light and converts its energy from light to heat. This heat can then be used to cut, coagulate, or actually vaporize blood vessels or tissue. In the latter case, the moisture within the body tissue is converted to steam and it literally dissipates into the air. Because the laser coagulates (seals off) blood vessels as they are cut, and because of its tremendous heat which sterilizes its target instantaneously, laser surgery is virtually bloodless and aseptic. It is a much quicker, less painful surgical procedure than hysterectomy, myomectomy, or even laparoscopy in that it does not require a single incision. (*Laparoscopy* involves the insertion of a fiberoptic scope through the abdomen to view the pelvic organs. See Chapter Four for additional information.) Patients may go home the same day and generally have a complete recovery in only a few days because far fewer complications can be expected to arise.

Various types of lasers have been used in gynecology for some time, including the "CO2" or carbon dioxide laser which will be discussed in Chapter Four on endometriosis. However, fairly new to the field are the use of the "Nd:YAG" (neodymium:yttrium aluminum garnet), "KTP" (potassium titanyl phosphate), and Argon lasers. While the latter two are employed in the treatment of endometriosis, the "YAG" laser can effectively treat the severe bleeding associated with fibroids. (See Figure 3.4.) This procedure is called *endometrial ablation.*

Laser Ablation of the Endometrium

You'll remember that in our discussion of fibroids earlier in the chapter, we said that the two most common symptoms that sufferers experience are hemorrhaging and pain. With laser ablation of the endometrium (lining of the uterus), a woman's bleeding can be markedly lessened or completely stopped *without ever having to remove her fibroids, let alone her uterus!*

After administering a general or regional anesthetic, a saline solution is used to enlarge the uterine cavity. Then, the laser specialist can employ the Nd:YAG beam to permanently destroy the offending tissue and blood vessels. The gynecologist has a clear view of the operative field via the hysteroscope, and is thus able to identify and sample any questionable areas.

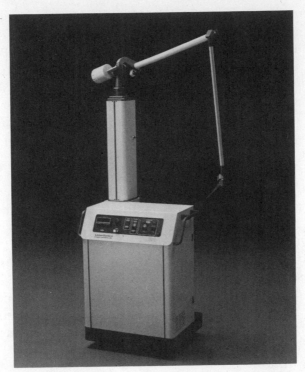

Figure 3.4   The "YAG" laser—One of several types of fiberoptic devices that concentrate and convert light energy into heat for cutting, coagulating, or vaporizing tissue.

Thus far this technique has been judged to be both safe and effective. Because the laser only penetrates to a known, controlled depth within the lining of the uterus, it cannot accidently burn too deeply, damaging any surrounding organs, such as the bladder or the intestine. Furthermore, in eight years of performing these procedures, there have been few instances where women required any additional procedures due to a recurrence of their symptoms.

However, there are women who cannot utilize this technique to cure their bleeding problems. It must be emphasized that this procedure *permanently destroys the endometrium* thus effectively sterilizing the woman who has it done. Therefore, it is *not* an option for women who still want to have children.

In addition, endometrial ablation is not appropriate for women who have suspicious tissue found when an initial sampling of their endometrium is taken on diagnostic hysteroscopy. This is to help put to rest one potential, but important theoretical complication of endometrial ablations. That is, the theoretical concern that a woman who has had her blood vessels destroyed, but who develops an endometrial cancer, will not bleed from that cancer. Bleeding is an important symptom of cancer, and one neither the patient nor the gynecologist would want to eliminate. Think of the analogy of a patient who is developing abdominal pain on her right side. The last thing a doctor wants to do is to give that patient potent pain-killers to mask her pain and hence possibly cause him to miss a rupturing appendix!

Again, it is important to emphasize that while laser specialists are concerned about, and recognize this potential problem, in reality, there has never yet been a single case of missed uterine cancer due to endometrial ablation. In fact, one might also theoretically argue (again, this has never been proven) that because women who have undergone ablations have less endometrium, they have less chance of developing endometrial cancer! Nevertheless, it is my opinion that a woman with endometrial cancer will *still* bleed, even after ablation, and that if yearly exams demonstrate that her uterine cavity has not inadvertently sealed off thus blocking the exit of blood through the vagina, she will be aware of that very significant symptom.

Finally, women who have pain along with their bleeding, and/ or women whose uterine cavities have become enlarged (due to the presence of large or multiple fibroids, increased growth and stretching of muscle fibers, and hormonal influences), will not have great success with endometrial ablation. (*Remember:* These procedures are primarily for the woman who is past childbearing, whose uterus is not greatly enlarged [less than 10 centimeters], and for whom bleeding is more significant than pain.) For women with much more severe symptoms and a much larger uterus (greater than 15 centimeters), another surgical technique has been developed out of a modification of an instrument used in urology called the *resectoscope.*

Electrocoagulation via the Resectoscope

When a woman has one or more fibroids growing into the uterine cavity, or pushing into the cavity like the tip of an iceberg, that have been causing her pain and bleeding, she may find that undergoing resectoscopy is the answer to her problems. Like endometrial abla-tion, this procedure begins with the insertion of the hysteroscope to directly visualize the uterine lining. Then, again like the laser procedures, the cavity is enlarged with fluid. Next, the resectoscope is used to shave the endometrium and sculpt out any fibroid tumors so that these areas are now flush with the remainder of the lining. In a woman who wishes to attempt pregnancy, this procedure has the advantage that it does not have to cause total scarring of the uterus. Thus the patient may have normal menstrual periods for several years after the removal of her fibroids without having to undergo abdominal surgery, and can go on to have a child as well. However, like any form of myomectomy, permanent results cannot be guaranteed. So, for a woman who is not concerned with her fertility, the resectoscope procedure may be taken one step further and used to electrically coagulate the entire endometrium, with the same end results as the laser.

The jury is still out on whether resectoscopy with electrocoagu-lation or laser ablation will ultimately prove the best method for eliminating the heavy bleeding associated with fibroids. For now, I choose to use the former with my patients who have large uterine cavities and more extensive symptoms, and the latter for those women with smaller cavities. Both are safe, simple, long-term alter-natives to open abdominal surgery for women with submucosal or intrauterine fibroids. Both result in the complete elimination of menstrual periods for at least half of all women, with the vast majority of the rest experiencing, if nothing else, normal, manage-able monthly menstrual cycles until they reach menopause.

Vaginal Myomectomy: A New Approach to an Old Idea

Earlier, myomectomy was introduced as an alternative to hysterec-tomy in which only the fibroids are removed, leaving the healthy portion of the uterus intact. However, women having this proce-dure must still face the risks and inconveniences of abdominal surgery, including blood loss, infection, general anesthesia, and a long postoperative recovery period. Now, several gynecologists re-move accessible intrauterine fibroids through the cervix and vagina. This is especially reserved for myomas with some degree of a pedicle (or stalk).

Fibroids: A Self-Help Guide

Symptoms to Look For...

- Heavy menstrual periods (using more sanitary napkins or tampons than you normally use, or having to use two pads or tampons at once).

- Passage of blood clots.

- Prolonged menstrual periods (lasting longer than previous menstrual periods, for example, seven instead of four days).

- Painful menstrual periods; the pain may be dull and aching or sharp and intense; it may not respond to the usual drugs prescribed for menstrual cramps.

- A sensation of heaviness in your lower abdomen, lower back or legs.

- Frequent or painful urination; the inability to control urinary flow.

- Dizziness, weakness, pallor; fainting spells.

- Problems conceiving or carrying a pregnancy to term.

What to Ask Your Doctor if He Tells You that You Have Fibroids...

- How did he arrive at that diagnosis? (It should have been made via a pelvic examination with ultrasound confirmation and measurements, not merely based on listening to your symptoms.)

- How large are they and are they likely to cause problems in terms of fertility? Women concerned with conceiving have a different outlook than women primarily concerned with avoiding surgery. (Remember that not all fibroids cause symptoms and some can be safely left alone.)

- What does he suggest the next course of therapy be (if any is necessary)?

What to Ask if Your Doctor Suggests Surgery...

- What type of surgery does he have in mind and why?
  - If you are having abnormal bleeding and your doctor suggests a D&C, ask how this will solve the fibroid problem and what his next step would be if the bleeding returns? Ask if he performs hysteroscopy in addition to D&C. If not, find someone who does.
  - If your doctor suggests myomectomy, ask if the fibroids are likely to recur before menopause, and how the myomectomy will be performed (traditional open abdominal route, vaginal route, laser

procedure)? Opt for a surgeon who uses the most modern, least invasive procedure.

- If your doctor suggests hysterectomy, determine his reasons for choosing such a radical approach (especially if he does so for mild or moderate disease or before other, less invasive procedures have been tried). *Always seek a second opinion!*

- How soon does the surgery need to be performed?

- What are the consequences if you decide not to have the surgery?

- How long will you need to be in the hospital (if at all)?

- How long will you need to recover at home before you can resume your normal activities?

- What are the short- and long-term side effects of the procedure?

- What are the risks associated with this surgery?

- How many of these operations has your doctor performed?

- What is the fee for this procedure and will your medical insurance cover the charges?

- Are there medical alternatives for shrinking the fibroids or amelioriating the symptoms?

What to Ask if Your Doctor Suggests Medical Therapy...

- How does this medication work?

- What are the potential side effects?

- Will this medication interact with other medications you may be taking?

- Is it contraindicated because you have other chronic medical problems?

- How effective is this medication?

- How long does the medication take to start working?

- Are the effects of the medication permanent?

- How long will you have to take the medication?

- Can it be self-administered?

- What are the costs?

- Will it influence your ability to become pregnant?

- What happens if you become pregnant while taking this medication?

Be a Smart "Shopper"...

- You should feel comfortable with your doctor. Remember, these are crucial, sometimes lifelong decisions you two are deciding. You should feel that you were not rushed, that you were treated as an individual, that the doctor listened to your questions and concerns, and that he addressed them to your satisfaction. Make sure you feel at ease in his office and with his staff.

- Always seek a second opinion for a serious problem or when surgery is suggested. It stands to reason that a second opinion should come from an independent physician who has no relation to your doctor.

- Be wary of a doctor who paints too rosy a picture—one that seems unrealistic, who gives you absolute guarantees, who seems cavalier about surgery and easily dismisses your problem, or the surgery, as "no big deal."

- Don't rush into major surgery unless you are convinced (by more than one doctor) that it is truly an emergency. Try to explore all of the alternatives first and attempt to preserve your uterus if you can.

First, using local anesthesia to numb the cervix, they insert several rods made of sterilized seaweed known as *laminaria*. Left in place overnight, the laminaria absorb fluid and swell, gently dilating the cervix. The next day, the laminaria are removed and a specialized grasping forceps is introduced through the cervix. It is attached to the fibroid and twisted, pulling the myoma loose, and removing it through the cervical os and out of the vagina.

This procedure is best accomplished with relatively small, submucosal fibroids and those that possess a stalk. Proper selection of patients minimizes the rare risk that the surgeon might damage the uterus or cause excessive bleeding.

Results of vaginal myomectomy compare favorably to the traditional abdominal approach. In one study by Dr. Ben-Baruch and his associates, bleeding was found to be much less, and hospitalization shorter (an average of 2.4 versus 7.8 days). In addition, in nearly 80 percent of patients followed for an average of over five years, no subsequent symptoms developed. In another investigation by Dr. Goldrath, vaginal removal of submucosal fibroids was successfully accomplished in 83 out of 92 women, with only 6 suffering complications (hemorrhage or uterine damage). The remaining nine women had fibroids that were too large to be removed in this manner. I have now become a disciple of Dr. Goldrath's technique and have found it to be extremely successful in well-selected patients.

Summary

Fibroids are the most common and troublesome gynecologic complaint of women. The pain and bleeding they cause lead millions of sufferers to undergo hysterectomy each year. Now we have specialized diagnostic and treatment techniques that can help a woman to preserve her uterus into menopause, when the symptoms of fibroids naturally abate from the withdrawal of estrogen.

Even significantly sized myomas can be safely managed by observation, as long as the fibroids do not cause excessive bleeding, and the patients do not wish to become pregnant. These women need only be carefully monitored with periodic pelvic exams and ultrasound. However, women whose myomas cause severe bleeding, pain, and a significantly enlarged, irregular uterus may require endometrial ablation and/or myomectomy as a permanent solution to the embarrassment, discomfort, and anemia associated with their monthly cycles. (One cautionary note must be added here. If other conditions are present in addition to the fibroids, myomectomy or ablation may not be the answer. This is especially true if adenomyosis is the problem, as we shall see in Chapter Four.)

This simple explanation is not meant to substitute for the highly individualized consideration each woman's case must be given in terms of choosing the treatment plan that is right for her. For some women, hysterectomy *is* the correct course, or it's the one that they desire. Others demand the minimal intervention that will solve their problem. *The number one job of the gynecologist is to address the patient's needs and desires, and put into perspective for her within the context of those needs and desires what her chance of success will be when availing herself of any particular plan of care.* Today, when so many alternatives are available and so much is known about the consequences of hysterectomy, if a gynecologist just says, "You don't need your uterus, let's take it out," his statements are both unwarranted and uncaring.

4

Endometriosis and Adenomyosis

I've rarely seen a fat woman with endometriosis. It's that type of individual who simply has to clean out the ashtrays all the time.

—Robert Kistner, M.D.

Endometriosis sufferers are defined with a plethora of observations about behavior, psychological makeup, and personality traits. The professionals making the observations . . . see women in pain, women anxious to have families, women who have had miscarriages, women who must make decisions about hysterectomies. . . . Most of the . . . statements from medical texts and interviews are buried in scientific language. They have an aura of authority and thus a ring of authenticity to them. Santa Claus is always round and jolly. Women with endometriosis are always trim and aggressive.

—Julia Older, 1984

It is an extremely rare person in this day and age who should ever need a hysterectomy for endometriosis, no matter how severe the condition. But this was not always the case. Consider Carol's situation:

Carol's symptoms began when she was in high school. Three or four days out of every month Carol would be bedridden with severe menstrual cramps. She felt helpless and frustrated—always wondering why she had been "singled out" to endure this agony. When Carol's school work began to suffer due to so much absenteeism, her mother took her to see a gynecologist. Carol's mother had endometriosis and she began to suspect that she had passed on this dreaded condition to her daughter. The doctor confirmed that Carol indeed had endometriosis and began hormonal therapy immediately. Unfortunately, Carol did not respond well to the medication, and her disease continued to progress. Exploratory surgery at age 25 revealed extensive endometriosis, with invasion of most of her pelvic organs. A short time later, she underwent a total abdominal hysterectomy with bilateral oophorectomy. While this finally put an end to her pain, Carol, now 44, is still very bitter about the experience. "I was never able to have children and, as a result, I feel I am lacking an experience that is an essential part of being a woman."

As we shall see, pain and infertility are a large part of the misery that accompanies endometriosis. Fortunately, the latest scientific advances in medicine and surgery can help women to overcome this common, invasive disorder.

Endometriosis: Still An Enigma

The first physicians and pathologists to describe endometriosis lived over 100 years ago, and the landmark papers still quoted today by many gynecologists were written in the 1920s by Dr. Sampson. Yet, many of the questions we have about endometriosis are as shrouded in mystery today as they were during the last century. For example, while we do have a working definition of endometriosis, we are still not completely sure as to what its cause is, or how it spreads (to areas as remote as the brain). Nor do we understand why *adenomyosis,* which is basically internal endometriosis, behaves so differently within the uterus from the way it does at remote sites, or why it afflicts a totally different group of women.

Simply defined, *endometriosis* is the presence of viable, proliferating endometrium outside its normal site, the lining of the uterus. Most commonly, the so-called glands and stroma that comprise the endometrium migrate to the ovaries and the fallopian tubes. The next most common sites (in descending order of incidence) include: the external surface of the uterus, the uterosacral ligaments (elastic fibers that connect the lower portions of the uterus to the sacrum), the area between the vagina and the rectum (called the rectovaginal septum), the cul-de-sac (the area behind the uterus), and the cervix, vulva, and vagina. However, endometriosis does not always limit itself to the pelvic cavity. Implants have been found in the large and small intestine, the bladder, the breasts, arms, legs, lungs, and even the brain! Just like the normal endometrium, they bleed cyclically every month. Thus they have been responsible for such bizarre and frightening symptoms in their unwitting sufferers as coughing up blood during the menstrual cycle (when implants are located in the lung, for instance).

When this aberrant tissue has enlarged to a size sufficient to categorize it as a tumor, it is called an *endometrioma*. Otherwise, the growths are simply known as implants. Because of its invasive nature and the bleeding it causes, endometrial tissue has frequently been mistaken for cancer. Although endometriosis may riddle the body with tumors, wreaking havoc on the various structures to which it metastasizes, endometriosis is neither cancerous nor precancerous. This is certainly reassuring, but it does not minimize the damage and discomfort endometriosis can cause.

The "Career Woman's Disease"? Causes and "Noncauses" of Endometriosis

A classic textbook description of the patient with endometriosis may be found in the 1986 edition of *Gynecology: Principles and Practices*, by Dr. Robert Kistner. Dr. Kistner was a pioneer in the treatment of endometriosis. In 1958 he introduced the use of hormonal therapy for this disease. Dr. Kistner states: "The median age of patients at the time of diagnosis is approximately 30 years. It is likely that endometriosis is more common in upper-middle-class professional women. Delayed and infrequent pregnancies may account for this association." Many gynecologists paint a similiar picture. Consider the experiences of one young woman, whom we shall call Joanne.

When Joanne was diagnosed, she felt she fit the picture perfectly. Joanne is a 35-year-old upper-echelon marketing executive who was recently married and is living in Manhattan. Joanne suffered for several years with dysmenorrhea and pain during intercourse. She managed to find expert medical care, and a combination of medication and laser surgery has reversed her disease to a large extent.

Yet, she's very distressed about what she perceives as the syndrome of "blaming the victim" that occurs with endometriosis. Says Joanne, "The first gynecologist I saw told me that I had endometriosis, the "career woman's disease." He implied that I had developed it because I was pursuing a career instead of being home raising a family. This was before I had even met Rick, my husband. He made me feel guilty that I hadn't married young and become pregnant right away, as if this had even been an option for me."

In fact, endometriosis is found in approximately 5 to 15 percent of all women aged 25 to 35 who undergo exploratory surgery for other causes, and in anywhere from 30 to 45 percent of infertile women undergoing laparoscopy as part of their diagnostic work-up. (More will be said about laparoscopy later in this chapter.) However, it is now known that the symptoms and pathology begin much earlier in life (usually in the teen years) for many women. The principal symptom, severe menstrual cramping, may be written off by parents and physicians as psychological, or as an adolescent attention-getting device. And it may be that the reason endometriosis is frequently diagnosed in upwardly mobile, educated career women is that they have the resources to seek sound medical care. Finally, much of the evidence about pregnancy ameliorating the disease is anecdotal. Many sufferers *have* had children, and may have found that the endometriosis further complicated both their disease and their pregnancy. Furthermore, the often-quoted low-pregnancy rates among endometriosis patients may be a consequence, not a cause, of the disease.

In fact, endometriosis is found in women of all ages, races, socioeconomic groups and occupations. It has been diagnosed in women who have had several children as well as in women who have never been pregnant.

Putting aside demographic characteristics, there may be some *menstrual* characteristics that women with endometriosis share. A large study conducted by Daniel Cramer and his associates involving over 4,000 women revealed that "women with short-cycle lengths (less than or equal to 27 days) and longer flow (greater than or equal to 1 week) had more than double the risk for endometriosis compared with women with longer cycle lengths and shorter duration of flow." These women also tended to have begun menstruating at a younger age, and to report greater menstrual pain. The latter finding may be one of the characteristics the authors admit may be a "consequence" rather than a "precursor" to the disease. In any case, it is still helpful in identifying high-risk patients. The authors conclude that the ". . . risk for endometriosis may relate to menstrual factors that predispose to greater pelvic contamination with menstrual products and to constitutional factors that influence endogenous hormonal levels." Here, they are probably alluding to another interesting finding in their investigation. They noted that long-term heavy smokers and strenuous exercisers are less likely to develop endometriosis. (This is just an epidemiologic fact. Obviously, I am not advocating this behavior as prevention or therapy for endometriosis!)

The study's findings that a shorter, less painful cycle results in less endometriosis dovetails with a more recent report in *Obstetrics and Gynecology* by Kirshon and Poindexter looking at the effects of various contraceptive methods on endometriosis. As one might expect, former users of intrauterine devices (more commonly known as IUDs) had a significantly higher rate of endometriosis than did women who took birth control pills. The IUD is known to cause longer, heavier, and more painful periods. It is also documented to cause an inflammatory reaction within the uterus. (This, in fact, may be one of its mechanisms of action in preventing pregnancy.) The Pill, however, thins out the endometrium and thus periods tend to be short and scant. This relative presence or absence of heavy bleeding leads us to explore the first, and perhaps the most popular, theory as to the true underlying cause of endometriosis.

Retrograde Menstruation

Normally, at the time of menstruation, the cervix relaxes and the uterus contracts to expel the endometrial lining that has built up during that particular cycle. Just the opposite scenario is believed to occur in women with endometriosis. In other words, the lower portion of the cervix goes into spasm, impeding the egress of blood out of the vagina. Instead, the blood is forced upward through the uterus and out the oviducts. Eventually, it winds up in the pelvic cavity where it can deposit around the fallopian tubes, and ovaries, or it can fall by gravity to the bottom of the pelvis and remain near the rectum or in the cul-de-sac. This so-called *retrograde menstruation* has been observed on numerous occasions when laparoscopies were performed on menstruating women. These endometrial "seedlings" then adhere to their surrounding structures and behave just as they would within the uterus: bleeding every month during menstruation. These bleeding adhesions may cause serious problems, as we shall see in the section dealing with the symptoms of endometriosis. Like the authors of the preceding two scientific investigations, Cramer, Kirshon, and Poindexter, many physicians believe that the heavier the menstrual flow, the greater the opportunity for endometrial implants to develop.

With the theory of retrograde menstruation we are still left with some of the "enigmas" of endometriosis. For example, why is retrograde menstruation observed in many more women than actually develop the disease? And, if endometrium escapes into the pelvic cavity during retrograde menstruation, how does this explain the "renegade" tissue that has been found in such mysterious places as under the arm or within the spinal column? The next theory has been proposed to explain this latter phenomenon.

Blood-Borne and Lymphatic Spread

The human body has two complex systems of transporting materials throughout its structure. The first and more familiar is the blood circulation. It is primarily responsible for carrying vital oxygen to the tissues that comprise our organ systems and for removing the waste products they generate. The blood also contains antibodies and specialized blood cells that gear up the immune response whenever the body is threatened by a foreign invader, such as a virus, bacteria, or allergen.

Like the bloodstream, the lymphatic system is vital to the body's immunologic defenses. In addition, it comprises a network of collecting vessels, channels, and organs that pepper the landscape of our bodies with the mission of collecting excess fluid that has escaped from the cells, tissues, organs, and blood vessels. It is possible that endometrial tissue infiltrates these two circulatory systems and is thus carried to remote and improbable sites of the body where it implants.

Hypotheses to explain endometriosis abound, and ultimately it may be discovered that there is a multifactorial cause. The following are a few of the other theories that have been advanced.

Coelomic Metaplasia

The term *metaplasia* refers to the differentiation of cellular material. It has been suggested that certain tissue may retain its ability to differentiate into other tissue under certain circumstances.

A fetus starts as a small ball of somewhat indistinct cells, but develops embryologically into the various complex organ systems of the newborn. What if the cells of the peritoneum, originally made up of *coelomic epithelium* during the fetal stage of a woman's development, retained their ability to transform in the presence of certain stimulants? Specifically, what if menstrual products (as from retrograde menstruation) and/or hormones (estrogen and progesterone) could trigger the development of endometrial tissue where it would not normally be present?

This is the crux of the metaplasia theory, first described by Drs. Meyer and Ivanoff at around the same time Dr. Sampson was proposing his notion of retrograde menstruation. One very intriguing aspect to this theory is that it alone accounts for the rare instances when endometriosis develops in the *absence* of menstruation. Approximately 5 percent of cases occur in postmenopausal women, usually when they have been taking estrogen supplements. Likewise, the literature cites very rare reports of endometriosis in women who have *never* menstruated, and in *men* receiving estrogen treatments for prostatic disease. The common denominator here is estrogen administered from an external source which may be the trigger for the induction of metaplasia.

Genetic, Immunologic, and Iatrogenic Factors

Your genetic background and/or the skill of your physician could have an effect on your risk of developing endometriosis and on your ability to control the extent of the disease! In his text, Dr. Droegemueller discusses the work of Dr. Simpson and his colleagues which revealed the presence of endometriosis in the close relatives (mothers or sisters) of patients seven times more frequently than in normal subjects. In addition, women with a genetic predisposition are found to develop the disease earlier in life, and to a greater extent than do women without fellow sufferers within the family.

One or more immunologic defects may explain why some women are particularly prone to endometriosis, according to Dr. Dmowski. Women with endometriosis seem to produce high titers of antibodies against their own endometrial tissue. This may be one factor that somehow plays a role in the development of the disease. Another may be an abnormality in the body's immune response that fails to destroy wayward endometrial tissue as it normally would. A final theory has to do with the role of prostaglandins (chemical substances that aid in the immune response). An excess of prostaglandins among women with endometriosis may be responsible for both the implants themselves and the severe cramping sufferers are known to endure.

Finally, endometriosis may be spread during the course of abdominal surgery, cesarean section, or laparoscopy. Implants have commonly been found at the sites of surgical scars and adhesions. However, as we shall see, improved operative techniques including laser surgery markedly reduce the incidence of physician-induced, or iatrogenic, endometriosis.

The Hallmarks of Endometriosis

"I couldn't concentrate on anything some days, the pain was so bad," confides Rochelle, a graduate student in clinical psychology. "I couldn't study or do my research. When I was interviewing clients, my mind was not focused on their problems. I'm the kind of person who's always on the move, involved with one project or another. Yet, when I had my period, my husband would come home and find me lying in bed waiting for the latest round of painkillers to take effect. . . .

I suspected that I might have endometriosis. We read that pregnancy might put this into remission so we began trying to have a baby. Months passed. The harder we tried, the greater was the tension between us. For one thing, it was painful for me to have intercourse in certain positions. We went to see my gynecologist who wanted to rule out other potential problems. All of the charting of my menstrual cycles and the battery of medical tests made sex more like a chore than a pleasure. Trying to conceive became a competition. It was us against this biological foe, endometriosis."

Pain

The symptom that is almost always associated with endometriosis is pain. This pain commonly takes one or both of these forms: dysmenorrhea (painful menses) and dyspareunia (pain during lovemaking). However, throughout this chapter we have been discussing the enigmas associated with endometriosis and here is yet another. Drs. Kistner, Droegemueller and others have documented on numerous occasions that the more extensive the disease, the less severe are the symptoms and vice versa. I personally have seen a pelvis containing large or extensive implants that do not cause the woman any discomfort, while another woman with only mild disease may be in excruciating pain. (Of course, this is not always the case, and the extent of pain is not a reliable measure of the degree of endometriosis.)

In addition to pelvic pain, women with implants located in sites outside of the pelvis will experience symptoms related to the organ that has been affected. For instance, implants located within or near the gastrointestinal tract may cause backache, abdominal tenderness, constipation, and pain and bleeding with bowel movements. Urinary tract disease may be associated with pain or pressure over the bladder, and the presence of discomfort or bleeding with urination. The rare woman unfortunate enough to have endometriosis within the chest may cough up blood or experience chest pain and shortness of breath.

The pain characteristic of endometriosis is *cyclic.* It is caused by the swelling and discharge of endometrial glands into the surrounding structures that it invades causing a local inflammatory response mediated by prostaglandins. Unlike so-called primary dysmenorrhea, which is pain during menstruation without any obvious underlying pathology, the secondary dysmenorrhea of endometriosis usually starts a few days before the actual menstruation and lasts longer into the cycle.

Dyspareunia, another characteristic of endometriosis, probably arises from direct pressure on endometrial implants that are low in the pelvis as well as from the inability of the pelvic organs to move freely during lovemaking. Often the endometriosis creates adhesive bands of tissue that bind structures. When these adhesions impede the ovaries and fallopian tubes, fertility is generally affected.

Infertility

Simply defined, infertility is the inability to conceive after one year of unprotected intercourse. Entire volumes have been written about the role of endometriosis in infertility because it has been estimated that anywhere from one-third to one-half of sterile women have endometriosis. In addition, these women have three times the risk of having a miscarriage if they do succeed in becoming pregnant.

As we mentioned, endometriosis can cause the oviduct to lose its mobility. Once it is unable to wrap itself around the egg and suction it into its innermost portions, conception is unlikely to occur. Ectopic pregnancy may also result because of this blockage which prevents the ovum from reaching its destination within the uterus. Instead, implantation takes place within the fallopian tube.

Aside from those severe cases where laparoscopy reveals the presence of obvious endometriosis within the ovary or obstructing the fallopian tube, the relationship of endometriosis to infertility is again a mystery. Some of the theories that have been proposed, but never proven, blame hormonal imbalances, immunologic defects, and excess production of prostaglandins. And of course, dyspareunia decreases the opportunity for conception to occur.

Bleeding

Although internal bleeding is the principal cause of the scarring and pain associated with endometriosis, actual abnormal menstrual bleeding is only present in about 15 to 20 percent of sufferers. This is in stark contrast to fibroids where bleeding seems to be the major symptom that motivates women to seek treatment. If abnormal bleeding does occur with endometriosis, it is most common as spotting just prior to the onset of menses or heavier flow during the menses.

Endometriosis: A Self-Help Guide

Symptoms to Look For . . .

- Common:
  - Severe menstrual cramping
  - Painful intercourse
  - Infertility
  - Heavy menstrual periods or other change in menstrual flow

- Less common:
  - Pain in organs outside of the pelvic area that worsens during menstruation (e.g., backache, abdominal discomfort, chest pain)
  - Constipation; pain and bleeding with bowel movements
  - Frequent urinary tract infections; pain and bleeding with urination

Diagnosis and Treatment: The Standard Response

We've talked about those symptoms, principally pelvic pain and infertility, that raise the spectre of endometriosis for patients and their physicians. Once suspected, this diagnosis can be made on pelvic or rectal examination if the disease has progressed sufficiently. Tumors or nodules may be palpable on a bimanual examination of the ovaries or on a rectal exam of the uterosacral ligaments and rectovaginal septum. The ovaries may appear to be enlarged, and the affected areas may be tender to manipulation, especially when the examination is conducted during menstruation. However, sometimes more sophisticated methods are needed to confirm a case where the signs and symptoms are not as straightforward. In this instance, ultrasound and a diagnostic laparoscopy will almost always be undertaken.

Diagnostic Laparoscopy

Laparoscopy is a procedure that allows the surgeon to directly view your uterus, ovaries, and fallopian tubes without the necessity of major abdominal surgery. The laparoscope is a tube-shaped fiberoptic instrument that is introduced into the abdominal cavity via a small incision within the navel. (See Figure 4.1.) Like hystero-scopy, laparoscopy is ambulatory surgery with a minimal recovery period. It also requires the presence of a gas, carbon dioxide, which is instilled into the abdomen prior to the insertion of the laparoscope. This pushes other abdominal structures out of the viewing area so that the gynecologic organs may be clearly exam-ined. Since laparoscopy is performed under general or regional anesthesia, there is no discomfort during the operation. Afterward, there may be tenderness at the site where the scope was inserted and painful cramping under your ribs or in your shoulder from gaseous irritation of nerve tissue. This abates in a few days once the carbon dioxide is absorbed by your body. There are very few risks associated with laparoscopy, although, as with all surgery, there may be wound infections or anesthesia complications. In addition, accidental punctures of bowel or blood vessels may rarely occur as the laparoscope is inserted. Of course, the benefits to be reaped are the ability to identify and locate any endometrial implants.

In mild disease, these may appear to be tiny purple or red, "blueberry" or "raspberry," spots. They may also be said to resemble powder burns. (See Figure 4.2.) Large endometriomas within the ovary are often called chocolate cysts because of the characteristic

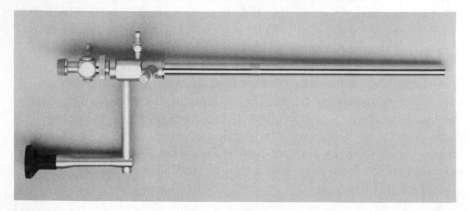

Figure 4.1   A laparoscope—A fiberoptic scope inserted via a minute incision in the abdomen and used to view the pelvic organs.

brownish appearance of the old blood that has accumulated within the tumor. (See Figure 4.3.) Finally, recent investigations have shown that many nonpigmented lesions in the pelvis previously overlooked are indeed areas of endometriosis as well!

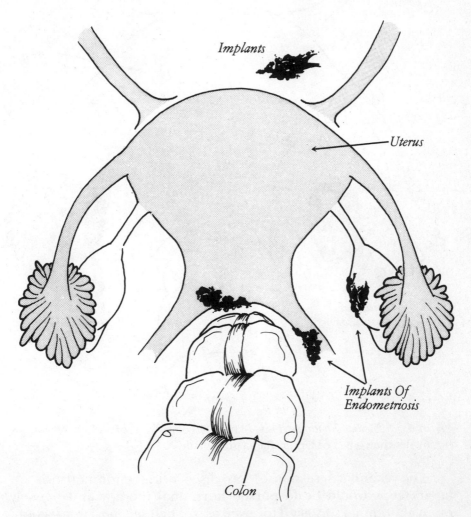

Figure 4.2   Mild endometriosis—Implants are small, flat patches of endometrial tissue growing outside of their normal location.

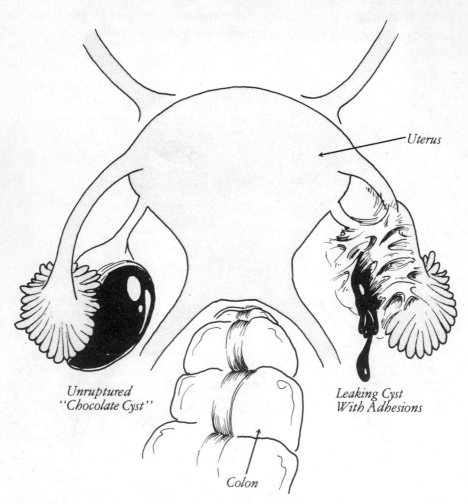

Figure 4.3   Moderate endometriosis—The "chocolate" cysts of endometriosis may be smaller than a pea or larger than a grapefruit.

The "standard response" on discovering endometriosis on laparoscopy would be to pursue hormonal therapy and possibly open abdominal surgery. However, as we shall see in a later section, through the combination of the laser and the laparoscope, women can now obtain immediate treatment in one simple procedure. First, let us explore the various treatment options offered by physicians following the "standard response."

Prevention as Treatment: "Be Fruitful and Multiply"

In Dr. Kistner's book, he very matter-of-factly states, "Early and frequent pregnancies appear to effectively decrease the frequency of endometriosis. . . ." Not only have we seen that this is a subject of controversy at the present time, but Dr. Kistner goes on to admit that ". . . this therapeutic strategy is incompatible with the life plans of most patients." Therefore, setting aside pregnancy as an unproven and inconvenient treatment modality, we move on to the next best thing—pseudopregnancy.

Pseudopregnancy: Can You Fool All of the Bodies All of the Time?

The use of oral contraceptive agents to reduce the severity of endometriosis was first introduced over 30 years ago. They work both as a means of birth control and in endometriosis by "fooling" a nonpregnant body into functioning as if it were pregnant. In other words, the constant presence of estrogen and progesterone from the pill disrupts the intricate hypothalamic-pituitary-ovarian axis preventing ovulation. Without ovulation, the lining of the uterus doesn't build up and shed. There is no menstruation and hence no activity by the ectopic endometrium. The accumulation of tissue, pain, swelling, and bleeding that regularly occur with endometriosis are averted.

Typically, to maintain this effect, a woman takes daily doses of estrogen and progesterone, with additional pills being added whenever any breakthrough bleeding occurs.

However, there are many medical contraindications to taking birth control pills, especially for older women. In addition, this therapy is replete with side effects. They include some very rare but serious ones such as the formation of blood clots in the brain, heart, or lung resulting in a stroke, heart attack, or pulmonary embolism. Less serious, but unpleasant side effects combined with only moderate efficacy cause many women to abandon this regimen. This was even truer in the early days of very high dose birth control pills than it is now. Thus, in response to the need for a "newer, better treatment," the drug Danazol was developed and approved by the FDA in 1975.

Danazol and Pseudomenopause

Menopause, the total cessation of menstruation, has been observed to be a definitive therapy for endometriosis. Of course, this process naturally occurs too late to help the majority of sufferers. Working with the model of menopause, researchers were able to develop a drug, called Danazol, which induces a simulated state of menopause known as *pseudomenopause* by reducing estrogen levels quite low.

Danazol is a derivative of the male hormone, testosterone. As we mentioned in Chapter Three, one of its drawbacks concerns its masculinizing side effects. It may also cause breakthrough bleeding (vaginal bleeding at other times of the month besides menstruation), headaches, or gastrointestinal side effects such as bloating. Danazol is also expensive, costing about $2.00 per tablet for name-brand (Danocrine) and about 30 percent less for generic forms. However, the major advantage is that Danazol, like oral contraceptives, allows for the control of endometriosis without surgery.

Danazol binds to the body's progesterone and androgen receptor sites thus increasing the amount of freely circulating testosterone present in a woman's system. Via another mechanism, Danazol also increases the metabolism of estrogen and progesterone. That is, they are broken down faster in the body and thus are less available to carry out their respective functions. Danazol has also been observed to decrease levels of gonadotrophin releasing hormone as well as ovarian hormone production. The end result of all of these effects is that ovulation and menstruation cease. The lining of the uterus as well as all of its associated ectopic implants atrophy. Again, as with the Pill, pain from swelling and bleeding temporarily or permanently stop.

Danazol is the only drug which has a beneficial effect on the antigen-antibody reaction that occurs in the peritoneal fluid (fluid in the abdominal cavity) of sufferers. By decreasing the antibodies present, Danazol decreases any destructive effect these antibodies exert on sperm thus theoretically enhancing a woman's fertility. In actuality, reducing antibody levels does not improve fertility, and women with endometriosis who take Danazol do not have a higher pregnancy rate than nonusers. Treatment is generally continued with Danazol for six months to a year, depending on a woman's response, her experience with side effects, other medical conditions that may be present, and her desire to become pregnant.

The "Definitive Therapy"

Dr. Kistner states: "For the patient older than 40 years with symptomatic endometriosis who has completed her family, the definitive therapy is total abdominal hysterectomy and bilateral oophorectomy." Likewise, "for the majority of patients with endometriosis involving organs outside the pelvis, total abdominal hysterectomy and bilateral oophorectomy are necessary." This is certainly "definitive therapy." In particular, removal of the ovaries precludes the proliferation of any existing or future endometrial implants. However, just as amputation of a leg will "cure" a severe infection and deformity that result from a motor vehicle accident, so may reconstructive surgery and intravenous antibiotics. The latter is obviously the more desirable choice.

As we've already mentioned, Dr. Kistner was until his recent untimely death a highly respected pioneer in the field of endometriosis. He had impeccable credentials. As such, he set an example for every local U.S. practitioner wanting to know the proper management of this condition. Yet, this statement of his concerning hysterectomy as definitive therapy for endometriosis represents the epitomy of the outdated and rigid attitudes and thought processes of American gynecologists. Perhaps when he first espoused this philosophy, adequate alternatives were not available and hence it was an appropriate therapeutic modality. However, times have changed and physicians should no longer take the easy way out for their patients. Every woman has the right to have her uterus preserved if she so desires, given all the options presently available.

You are probably reading this book because you wish to avoid hysterectomy if at all possible. And as we shall see, today's repertoire of medical and surgical techniques provide viable alternatives for many women. Despite this, *the only diagnosis for which hysterectomy increased between 1965 and 1984 according to a large-scale government study was endometriosis*. It not only increased—it skyrocketed by 176 percent! This is because the standard response for physicians has been major abdominal surgery either after a failed trial of hormonal therapy or in combination with hormonal therapy. Within their protocol, the abdomen is opened, explored, and any evident endometriosis is excised. If symptoms recur, the next step after laparotomy is extirpation of all the pelvic organs. As Dr. Kistner further advises, "Large bilateral ovarian endometrial cysts with extensive peritoneal endometriosis and numerous pelvic adhesions or marked invasion of the rectosigmoid and rectovaginal space constitute the most urgent indications for radical removal of all the pelvic organs, regardless of the age of the patient."

My approach to the treatment of endometriosis incorporates some of those methods employed in the "standard response," and expands on them. However, it deviates greatly in philosophy in that I believe that it is a rare woman who will wind up needing so-called "definitive" treatment. Today's treatment options are more extensive than ever, and they offer much hope to the woman experiencing the agonizing pain and infertility associated with this disease.

The Best Approach to Diagnosis and Treatment

Classifying the Disease

Treatment of endometriosis varies depending on the age of the woman and the extent of her disease. In an attempt to clarify the latter, several classification systems have been developed that divide endometriosis into stages. They all attempt to describe the extent of the disease from mild to severe by discussing the relative presence or absence of endometriomas, adhesions, and/or the involvement of organs outside the pelvic cavity. (See Figures 4.2, 4.3, and 4.4 and Table 4.1.) The American Fertility Society classification of endometriosis is probably one of the more widely used systems. (See Figure 4.5.) It assigns a number of points depending on laparoscopic findings. This system is an excellent method of scientifically quantifying endometriosis, but it unfortunately fails to capture the *qualitative* aspects to this disease. And it is the quality of a woman's life; the character of her pain and symptoms on which we must base therapy in the everyday practice of medicine. As with the standard response, pelvic examination, ultrasound and laparoscopy are key components to the diagnosis of endometriosis. (Staging is based on laparoscopic findings alone.) In addition, MRI (see Chapter Three) is proving helpful as it can scan the blood-filled cysts and fibrotic tissue that ultrasound and even CAT scans lack the specificity to identify.

In the next section, we briefly explore what is known about a new test that may hold a future key to the diagnosis of this disease—a blood test for endometriosis.

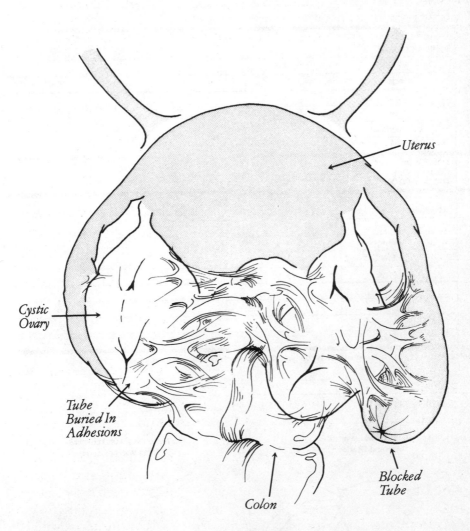

Figure 4.4 Severe endometriosis—In some cases, bands of fibrous scar tissues (adhesions) bind the pelvic organs together.

THE AMERICAN FERTILITY SOCIETY
REVISED CLASSIFICATION OF ENDOMETRIOSIS

Patient's Name _____ Date_____

Stage I   (Minimal) - 1-5
Stage II (Mild)   - 6-15
Stage III (Moderate) - 16-40
Stage IV (Severe)   - >40
Total_____

Laparoscopy_____ Laparotomy_____ Photography_____
Recommended Treatment_____

Prognosis_____

PERITONEUM	**ENDOMETRIOSIS**	<1cm	1-3cm	>3cm
	Superficial	1	2	4
	Deep	2	4	6
OVARY	R Superficial	1	2	4
	Deep	4	16	20
	L Superficial	1	2	4
	Deep	4	16	20

	POSTERIOR CULDESAC OBLITERATION	Partial	Complete
		4	40

	ADHESIONS	<1/3 Enclosure	1/3-2/3 Enclosure	>2/3 Enclosure
OVARY	R Filmy	1	2	4
	Dense	4	8	16
	L Filmy	1	2	4
	Dense	4	8	16
TUBE	R Filmy	1	2	4
	Dense	4*	8*	16
	L Filmy	1	2	4
	Dense	4*	8*	16

*If the fimbriated end of the fallopian tube is completely enclosed, change the point assignment to 16.

Additional Endometriosis: _____

Associated Pathology: _____

To Be Used with Normal
Tubes and Ovaries

L

R

To Be Used with Abnormal
Tubes and/or Ovaries

L

R

EXAMPLES & GUIDELINES

STAGE I (MINIMAL)

```
PERITONEUM
  Superficial Endo  –  1-3cm    - 2
R. OVARY
  Superficial Endo  –  < 1cm    - 1
  Filmy Adhesions   –  < 1/3    - 1
           TOTAL POINTS           4
```

STAGE II (MILD)

```
PERITONEUM
  Deep Endo         –  >3cm     - 6
R. OVARY
  Superficial Endo  –  < 1cm    - 1
  Filmy Adhesions   –  < 1/3    - 1
L. OVARY
  Superficial Endo  –  < 1cm    - 1
           TOTAL POINTS           9
```

STAGE III (MODERATE)

```
PERITONEUM
  Deep Endo         –  >3cm     - 6
CULDESAC
  Partial Obliteration          - 4
L. OVARY
  Deep Endo         –  1-3cm    - 16
           TOTAL POINTS          26
```

STAGE III (MODERATE)

```
PERITONEUM
  Superficial Endo  –  >3cm     -4
R. TUBE
  Filmy Adhesions   –  < 1/3    - 1
R. OVARY
  Filmy Adhesions   –  < 1/3    - 1
L. TUBE
  Dense Adhesions   –  < 1/3    - 16*
L. OVARY
  Deep Endo         –  <1 cm    -4
  Dense Adhesions   –  < 1/3    -4
           TOTAL POINTS          30
```

STAGE IV (SEVERE)

```
PERITONEUM
  Superficial Endo  –  >3cm     - 4
L. OVARY
  Deep Endo         –  1-3cm    - 32**
  Dense Adhesions   –  < 1/3    - 8**
L. TUBE
  Dense Adhesions   –  < 1/3    - 8**
           TOTAL POINTS          52
```

*Point assignment changed to 16
**Point assignment doubled

STAGE IV (SEVERE)

```
PERITONEUM
  Deep Endo         –  >3cm     - 6
CULDESAC
  Complete Obliteration         - 40
R. OVARY
  Deep Endo         –  1-3cm    - 16
  Dense Adhesions   –  < 1/3    - 4
L. TUBE
  Dense Adhesions   –  >2/3     - 16
L. OVARY
  Deep Endo         –  1-3cm    - 16
  Dense Adhesions   –  >2/3     - 16
           TOTAL POINTS         114
```

Determination of the stage or degree of endometrial involvement is based on a weighted point system. Distribution of points has been arbitrarily determined and may require further revision or refinement as knowledge of the disease increases.

To ensure complete evaluation, inspection of the pelvis in a clockwise or counterclockwise fashion is encouraged. Number, size and location of endometrial implants, plaques, endometriomas and/or adhesions are noted. For example, five separate 0.5cm superficial implants on the peritoneum (2.5 cm total) would be assigned 2 points. (The surface of the uterus should be considered peritoneum.) The severity of the endometriosis or adhesions should be assigned the highest score only for peritoneum, ovary, tube or culdesac. For example, a 4cm superficial and a 2cm deep implant of the peritoneum should be given a score of 6 (not 8). A 4cm deep endometrioma of the ovary associated with more than 3cm of superficial disease should be scored 20 (not 24).

In those patients with only one adnexa, points applied to disease of the remaining tube and ovary should be multipled by two. **Points assigned may be circled and totaled. Aggregation of points indicates stage of disease (minimal, mild, moderate, or severe).

The presence of endometriosis of the bowel, urinary tract, fallopian tube, vagina, cervix, skin etc., should be documented under "additional endometriosis." Other pathology such as tubal occlusion, leiomyomata, uterine anomaly, etc., should be documented under "associated pathology." All pathology should be depicted as specifically as possible on the sketch of pelvic organs, and means of observation (laparoscopy or laparotomy) should be noted.

Figure 4.5   The American Fertility Society worksheet for endometriosis—Frontside; backside shown on facing page.

Table 4.1 Classification of endometriosis

Stage	Points	Findings
I. Mild	1 to 5	Small, scattered, and superficial implants that do not involve the uterus or fallopian tubes; no scar tissue; small, infrequent ovarian implants; no endometriomas.
II. Moderate	6 to 15	Multiple, small endometriomas or implants on one or both ovaries; minimal scar tissue formation around the ovaries, fallopian tubes, or other involved sites.
III/IV. Severe/ Extensive	16 to 30/ 31 to 54	Large tumors of the ovary; extensive scarring with blockage of the fallopian tubes; wide-spread damage to other pelvic and abdominal structures, including bowel or bladder involvement.

Serum Calcium 125

Calcium 125 is an "antigen" or protein that has been found to be present in excessive amounts within the blood of 80 percent of women suffering from ovarian cancer. Elevated levels have also been noted in pregnant women and in women with other benign pelvic conditions. Most recently, work with this chemical marker has focused on its association with endometriosis. Numerous studies now reveal that the serum obtained from a woman with endometriosis is likely to contain higher levels of Calcium 125 than blood taken from a woman without the condition. More specifically, levels in these women are greatest during menstruation, but don't usually attain the values recorded when ovarian cancer is present. This allows a distinction to be made between cancer, endometriosis, and the absence of any pelvic pathology according to where blood levels fall along a scale.

At present, serum Calcium 125 levels are only in limited usage, primarily in diagnosing the recurrence of endometriosis in women who have already had diagnostic laparoscopy and treatment. This is because patients with mild disease have levels very similar to normal women. Thus far, abnormal elevations have only been recognized in women with severe disease (Stages III and IV, according to the American Fertility Society classification). However, in the future, this ability to differentiate minimal from extensive disease may assist the surgeon in deciding whether surgery is indicated, as well as when a second laparoscopy should be performed to explore a suspected resurgence in disease.

Treatment: At What Age and In What Stage?

The Teen Years

A woman may first experience the pain of endometriosis when she is an adolescent. At this point in her life, dysmenorrhea, more than fertility, is her prime concern. More than likely, she has minimal pathology and thus minimally invasive therapy may be the extent of any necessary intervention. Still, we must never lose sight of the fact that the seeds of her reproductive future may have already been sown.

A clinical diagnosis is often possible in a teenager who has never been sexually active by performing an abbreviated pelvic exam and by palpating the uterosacral ligaments for tenderness and swelling on rectal exam and by performing a diagnostic ultrasound. If these signs and symptoms are noted, we must begin management to relieve pain, and more important, to avert any future fertility problems.

Early on, all that may be necessary for pain management are the so-called nonsteroidal anti-inflammatory medications discussed in Chapter Three. These can reduce the painful effects of prostaglandins to a manageable level allowing young women with early endometriosis to resume their school life and social activities.

To prevent progression of their disease, I place my young patients on a therapeutic trial of birth control pills. As noted before, if endometriosis is at the root of their pain, these hormones will effectively shrink the implants causing a regression in symptoms. Likewise, if endometriosis has not as of yet invaded a teenager's body, she may still experience relief with the Pill if she has the precursor to endometriosis: retrograde menstruation. Remember that spasm of the uterus may force blood backward into the pelvic cavity eventually leading to pathology. Somehow, these hormones seem to diminish this painful spasm.

While I try to avoid surgery in adolescents, if a young woman does not respond to birth control pills, it then becomes necessary to resort to laparoscopy to search for the cause of her pain. And, as with women of any age, if laparoscopy reveals endometriosis, laser surgery should be performed right then and there.

The Reproductive Years

Once a woman displaying the symptoms of endometriosis reaches her reproductive years, it is necessary to become more aggressive in the diagnosis and treatment of her disease in order to safeguard her fertility. Specifically, laparoscopy should be performed—both to examine the extent of the disease and to initiate treatment via laser surgery when necessary.

The aim of treatment is to contain the spread of endometriosis and to prevent the destruction of the fallopian tubes and ovaries which would impede her ability to become pregnant. The availability of laser for use in conjunction with laparoscopy may afford the patient an immediate, complete, and low-risk alternative to laparotomy or lengthy courses of drug therapy. In 1988, Dr. Gordon Davis and Dr. Robert Brooks said of laser laparoscopy, "Vaporization and excision of endometriosis is almost always performed as an outpatient procedure, saving the patient both time and money. The morbidity of removal of endometriosis by laparoscopy is considerably less than that with laparotomy."

Laser Laparoscopy

Like the other women whose stories we have told in this chapter, Sherry coped with years of agonizing pain from endometriosis. She tells of being rushed by ambulance from her work place to the hospital one day because the nurse practitioner at the employee health department feared she had ruptured her appendix. In fact, the excruciating pain was from a large endometrioma located on her right side. Yet she coped as best as she could, making do with hormonal treatments and medications because Sherry was unwilling to subject herself to the major surgery she was told would be necessary to eradicate the disease from her body.

All of this changed when she began actively trying to get pregnant. She speaks of that time as being "rescued from an abyss of despair." Sherry decided to see a reproductive specialist who performed laser laparoscopy, excising 90 percent of the endometrial tissue (including a very large ovarian cyst), and repairing one damaged fallopian tube. Now, a year later, Sherry is pain-free and pregnant with her first child. Says Sherry, "I feel like life has started over for me."

Unlike laser ablation of the endometrium which uses the YAG laser focused through the hysteroscope, the CO_2 laser is preferred in the excision of endometriosis. This is because its beam may be aimed more precisely over the specific areas to be eliminated. (The newer KTP and argon lasers where available are even superior to the CO_2 laser because of their fiberoptic design and because they allow the surgeon to more deeply vaporize as well as excise the endometriotic lesions. These new lasers probably represent the wave of the future for laporoscopic surgery).

Laser laparoscopy has several advantages over traditional surgery. It safely vaporizes troublesome implants while cauterizing blood vessels. Less bleeding means better visualization of the operative field, less risk of the need for transfusion, and no need for suturing. As with endometrial ablation, the laser generates heat sufficient to sterilize the wound, cutting down on postoperative infections. But perhaps of most critical importance in endometriosis is that minimal scar tissue is produced during laser procedures. Since adhesions may be the sites of subsequent endometrial implants, such problems are averted in women who have undergone laser surgery. Finally, studies have revealed that laser laparoscopy is highly effective. In one such investigation of 158 women by Dr. Gordon Davis, he noted "Significant relief of dysmenorrea and dyspareunia as well as enhanced fertility. . . ." In this study, the surgery generally took about an hour and a half, with only four patients requiring hospitalization for observation and none requiring subsequent laparotomy.

After Surgery: What Next?

Unfortunately, neither traditional laparotomy nor modern laser techniques can guarantee a complete and permanent remission for all women. Sometimes, microscopic seedlings or atypical-appearing lesions are left behind. In my practice, I may institute medical therapy following laparoscopy to prevent the resurgence of any vestigial endometriosis. This depends on the degree of the endometriosis and whether the woman desires pregnancy at that time. (In the latter case, medications would be counterproductive.)

Besides oral contraceptives and Danazol, we may now call on an expanded menu of medications that may be rotated to suppress menstruation and ovulation until a woman is ready to become pregnant or until she enters menopause.

GnRH Agonists

The use of GnRH agonists in the treatment of endometriosis has been called a "medical oophorectomy" because it effectively shuts down ovarian function and induces a state of pseudomenopause. Many studies now report that laparoscopies performed on women who undergo therapy with these agents experience marked reduction in their implants. Both of these characteristics make GnRH agonists similar to Danazol therapy in some ways. GnRH agonists, however, do not demonstrate the androgenic side effects that 85 percent of women on Danazol complain of. There is no weight gain, acne, deepening of the voice, or hair growth. Perhaps more important, there seem to be no adverse effects on either the liver or on serum cholesterol levels: both of which are known to occur with Danazol.

But the fact that the effects of this drug are quickly reversible once it is discontinued is a double-edged sword. On the one hand, ovulation quickly resumes, allowing women to become pregnant almost immediately once their disease has been lessened or eradicated. It also means that the annoying anti-estrogenic side effects, such as hot flashes, decreased libido, and vaginal dryness, are short-lived. On the other hand, this reversibility means that the possibility of an exacerbation of the endometriosis is possible at any time once therapy is discontinued.

Tamoxifen and Megestrol Acetate

Tamoxifen is an anti-estrogen medication that may achieve this effect by competing with estrogen for binding sites in target tissues. In limited studies where this drug was administered to women unresponsive to other therapies, tamoxifen showed promise. It seemed to lessen symptoms and shrink implants without causing major side effects. Interestingly, tamoxifen does not always inhibit ovulation and menstruation. Thus one cautionary note must accompany this statement. Since a woman may become pregnant while taking this medication and its effects on the fetus are unknown, it would be wise for women to practice contraception until they have discontinued therapy.

Megestrol Acetate (Megace) is a powerful progestational drug currently used for the treatment of women with carcinoma of the breast or endometrium. Now it is being introduced as a second line endometriosis medication, meaning it is prescribed to maintain low estrogen levels and prevent cyclic menstrual bleeding and therefore prevent a recurrence of endometriosis in women under therapy who are not attempting pregnancy. Megace has few side effects except for occasional breakthrough bleeding. It is better tolerated but not as powerful as GnRH in suppressing estrogen.

Synthetic Estrogens and Progesterones

Diethylstilbestrol (DES) is a potent estrogen that gained notoriety a generation ago when it was observed that there was a significant increase in the incidence of vaginal cancer in the daughters of women who took this medication during their pregnancies to avert miscarriage. Now, at least two physicians, Drs. Lockhart and Karnaky, writing in the *American Journal of Obstetrics and Gynecology*, have advocated its return from banishment as a treatment for endometriosis, although what its mechanism of action would be is unclear. Presumably, it would compete with the body's natural estrogen for binding sites as does Tamoxifen. According to Drs. Lockhart and Karnaky, "Only diethylstilbestrol, properly given, can diagnose the disease without invasion, eradicate endometriotic cells and safely preserve fertility and femininity." This is a controversial area, and the truth of this statement remains to be seen.

Other physicians suggest the return of an old, no longer approved treatment: Medroxyprogesterone Acetate (MPA), which is otherwise known as "Provera" or "Depo-provera." This is a synthetic progesterone that inhibits the synthesis of gonadotrophins. While this medication does reduce signs and symptoms of endometriosis for some women, most physicians believe that more effective medications are now available and cause less side effects.

Both DES and MPA are mentioned here if only to make you aware of their existence, or to clarify information you may have heard about them. They are at this point not the preferred forms of therapy, although they may be used as interim measures.

Adenomyosis: Endometriosis Turned "Inside-Out"?

Margaret is a 52-year-old mother of three who was diagnosed as having multiple fibroid tumors several years ago. She had severe bleeding with her menstrual periods and developed an alarming iron deficiency anemia as a result. In addition, Margaret described the pains she had with her menses as reminiscent of labor contractions. She underwent a myomectomy and five fibroids were removed from her uterus. Needless to say, Margaret was shocked and dismayed when the surgery failed to have any influence on her pain. It turned out that, in addition to the fibroids, Margaret had adenomyosis.

Adenomyosis is also known as internal endometriosis. But this term is only remotely correct in that both endometriosis and adenomyosis are comprised of endometrial glands and stroma present in an abnormal location. This is where the similarities end. Indeed, endometriosis and adenomyosis overlap in only 20 percent of women. Furthermore, adenomyosis more often afflicts middle-aged women (aged 40 to 50) who have had several children. In contrast, the most common picture of the endometriosis sufferer is a childless woman in her twenties or thirties.

In adenomyosis, as in endometriosis, the most common symptom is dysmenorrhea. Again, there is ectopic endometrium present, but instead of being located outside the womb, it actually invades the myometrium of the uterus itself. Adenomyosis does not seem to proliferate and bleed cyclically with menstruation as dramatically as does endometriosis. Instead, this aberrant tissue causes a generalized *hypertrophy* or enlargement of the uterine muscle fibers with subsequent overall growth of the uterus. The uterus takes on a generalized tender and spongy nature. Because of this enlargement as well as the pain and occasional abnormal bleeding adenomyosis can cause, it is sometimes mistaken for fibroids.

In actuality, a definitive diagnosis is difficult to make and it is often only discovered after hysterectomy when pathologists examine the uterine tissue that has been removed. Pelvic exam may reveal an enlarged, spongy uterus. Ultrasound and laparoscopy occasionally reveal adenomyosis as well. In addition, MRI is showing promise in detecting adenomyosis as well as in differentiating it from leiomyomas.

In addition to lacking a method of definitive diagnosis for adenomyosis, physicians also lack a definitive form of therapy. For example, adenomyosis has been poorly responsive to hormonal therapy. This may be because, unlike its external counterpart, adenomyosis seems to be deficient in hormone receptors. Occasionally, superficial adenomyosis with abnormal bleeding as its major symptom may be helped by an endometrial ablation.

Fortunately, the majority of women with adenomyosis are without symptoms. Unfortunately for those who do suffer its most serious effects, hysterectomy may be their only recourse.

Summary

We have seen that endometriosis and adenomyosis rarely need to result in hysterectomy—the former because of the availability of a wide variety of new, less radical treatment options, and the latter because it rarely causes severe enough symptoms to necessitate such extreme measures. Yet, this does not minimize the detrimental effects endometriosis can impose on women, especially when it strikes during the prime of their careers and reproductive years.

Fortunately, most cases of endometriosis may be successfully managed using a combination of medical and surgical therapies.

Women may now undergo one laparoscopic procedure to simultaneously diagnose and treat their disease. Followed up by a combination and/or rotation of analgesics and various suppressive hormonal preparations, their endometriosis may remain in remission for an indefinite period. This permits 90 percent of women to avoid more extensive traditional surgery including the "routine" initial diagnostic laparoscopy with follow-up laparotomy. The minority of women who do require open abdominal surgery are those whose disease has caused extensive invasion of the bowel. While it is important to note that most times intestinal endometrial scar tissue can be safely separated from the pelvic organs using the laparoscope, most physicians agree that laparoscopic laser surgery is not feasible if the endometriosis is deeply embedded in the bowel wall.

Although endometriosis continues to present us with challenges and enigmas, we continue to progress to less invasive and more effective means of helping women to cope with this, one of the most dreaded "benign" diseases.

5

Hormonal Imbalance and Dysfunctional Uterine Bleeding

When the patient is aged more than 40 years, and when the haemorrhage fails to respond to more simple measures, hysterectomy is often indicated. It is the treatment of choice in all cases of persistent or recurrent postmenopause bleeding for which there is not an obvious cause. Hysterectomy can usually be carried out easily by the vaginal route and this involves little risk and upset.

—*Sir Norman Jeffcoate,*
Jeffcoate's Principles of Gynaecology, 1987 edition

In Chapters Three and Four we discussed two of the most common *organic* conditions that result in hysterectomy—fibroids and endometriosis. However, at some point in their lives, many women experience abnormal uterine bleeding for which no definite pathology can be found and this occasionally can lead to thoughts of hysterectomy. Certainly, copious and erratic vaginal bleeding can be a very frightening symptom and might seem a very logical reason to have an urgent hysterectomy. As we shall see, this is not necessarily the case. In fact, there may be no need for surgery of any kind. But before going any further, it is necessary to understand exactly what is happening when a woman suddenly experiences abnormal uterine bleeding.

A Lesson in Physiology

The term *abnormal uterine bleeding* is often confused with *dysfunctional uterine bleeding*. It's important to distinguish between these two conditions. Abnormal uterine bleeding is not a disease; it is a symptom that may signal any one of many different diseases. In fact, *Jeffcoate's Principles of Gynaecology* lists over 30 causes of abnormal uterine bleeding ranging from infections to cancer to heart failure. This is important to remember because it is necessary for the gynecologist, when confronted with a woman who has experienced unexpected vaginal bleeding, to consider her entire physiologic make-up and not merely her pelvic organs. For instance, it may be that a woman's sudden bleeding episodes are as a result of a disorder of her hematologic system which interferes with blood clotting, or they may be from a thyroid condition that has altered her metabolism.

Once these disease states have been ruled out, a hormonal imbalance is most likely to blame. This diagnosis of exclusion is called dysfunctional uterine bleeding. In other words, dysfunctional uterine bleeding results when there is a disturbance in the normal, cyclical production of hormones by the ovary which may or may not interfere with ovulation. This then causes a change in the pattern, duration, or amount of the menstrual flow. It is not as a result of another organic cause.

You will recall that every month, a woman releases chemical messengers from her brain signaling the ovary to ready an egg for fertilization. Simultaneously, several follicles housing ova mature, but only one ultimately ruptures. This is called the *follicular* phase. At the same time, within the uterus, the endometrium is in its *proliferative* stage, readying itself for implantation should this egg be fertilized. Once the egg is released at ovulation, the ovary enters the *luteal* phase and the empty follicle becomes a corpus luteum, producing estrogen and progesterone. Within the uterus, the endometrium is now *secretory,* meaning it is producing nutrients in preparation for sustaining life if pregnancy is inevitable. If not, hormone levels decline and the lining breaks down resulting in menstruation.

For those of you who are experiencing irregular bleeding, the next sections are a bit technical, but please bear with me, because they will explain how and why this bleeding comes about.

Dysfunctional Bleeding: The Short Menstrual Period

Sometimes, the ovary goes through its normal cycle, but it does so at an accelerated pace. The follicular phase speeds up for a variety of reasons as does the proliferation of the endometrium and menstruation takes place every two to three weeks instead of the usual four to five weeks. This type of dysfunctional uterine bleeding causes more frequent periods without any alteration in the amount of the flow. It may occur after pregnancy while the pituitary is still readjusting or when any kind of physical or psychological stress influences the nervous system and its subsequent production and release of hormones. Usually, this form of dysfunctional uterine bleeding resolves on its own in a few months and is no cause for concern.

The Abnormal Corpus Luteum

Another type of dysfunctional uterine bleeding can occur when ovulation again takes place normally. However, after the normal release of the egg, the "shell" that remains, called the corpus luteum, doesn't function as it should. This condition usually causes heavier, more prolonged periods that come at their *normal* time. A defect in the corpus luteum in some ways fails to properly produce progesterone and the endometrium breaks down erratically. While difficult to diagnose, if an endometrial biopsy is performed (to be explained later on), it will reveal an improperly matured uterine lining due to inadequate progesterone. This is more often than not an isolated event. Once the aberrant corpus luteum ceases its activity and the next cycle begins, a woman usually resumes her normal menstrual pattern. Again, treatment is usually unnecessary unless this tends to happen on a regular basis.

Anovulatory Bleeding

Seventy percent of women with dysfunctional uterine bleeding are at the extremes of their menstrual life, and 70 percent of women with dysfunctional bleeding are also "anovulatory"; in other words, they do not ovulate. These statistics coincide for good reason as women most frequently have erratic ovulation either when they are first beginning to menstruate or when they are approaching menopause.

In some forms of anovulatory dysfunctional uterine bleeding, a follicle ripens but no egg is released. Instead, the ovum dies and remains within the follicle, sometimes turning into an ovarian cyst. The ovary produces estrogen, but because there is no ovulation, no progesterone is secreted. This is important because it interferes with the normal functioning of the feedback mechanism which sends signals to the brain to stop estrogen production. Estrogen that is unopposed by progesterone will continue to be manufactured, causing a build-up of the uterine lining that may continue for weeks, until the estrogen-producing "granulosa" cells of the ovary literally burn out, like a dying battery. When this finally happens, and when the lining of the uterus has become so thick that the amount of estrogen naturally produced cannot maintain it, the endometrium will begin to break down. A woman who has had no bleeding for perhaps six weeks while estrogen has been building and supporting an unusually heavy lining (called a *hyperplastic endometrium*) now starts to bleed heavily. This hemorrhaging may continue steadily or erratically for anywhere from two to eight weeks and can cause serious complications, such as life-threatening anemias.

Interestingly, unlike the severe bleeding that may accompany other gynecologic conditions, such as ectopic pregnancies or serious infections, dysfunctional uterine bleeding is usually *painless*, thus providing an important diagnostic clue. Dysfunctional or anovulatory bleeding must be differentiated from other more serious conditions such as submucosal fibroid. Serious problems such as endometrial cancer can present in the same manner. Therefore, diagnostic evaluation by hysteroscopy and biopsy is crucial. Dysfuctional uterine bleeding can occur as a result of any disturbance in a woman's physical or emotional state. So delicately in tune are mind and body, that menstrual cycles can be altered by physical illness, marital or job-related pressures, alterations in nutritional state resulting in either weight gain or loss—even "good" stress like travel abroad or moving into a new home. But regardless of the underlying cause, dysfunctional uterine bleeding deserves prompt identification (through the elimination of other pathologic conditions) and intervention to both stop the immediate hemorrhaging and to prevent a recurrence.

A Diagnosis of Exclusion

As we've already emphasized, bleeding that appears to be from the uterus may stem from a variety of underlying causes, some of which may not even arise from the genital tract. For example, aside from those disease states elsewhere in the body that may disrupt menstruation, a woman may perceive that she is having vaginal bleeding when the source may be a bladder infection or a hemorrhoid. Because a woman's urethra, vagina, and rectum are in close proximity, it is easy to become confused. Careful documentation of the source of the bleeding via a thorough history and physical examination including Pap smear are the first step in establishing the nature of the bleeding. Sometimes, as when the bleeding is a one-time event, careful observation may be all that is necessary. If the problem seems persistent, then a physician may order a battery of laboratory tests to check for bleeding disorders, endocrine imbalances, or pregnancy. Occasionally, hysteroscopy or laparoscopy may be undertaken in trying to determine the source of abdominal bleeding. But perhaps the most crucial test in definitively establishing the existence of dysfunctional uterine bleeding is a simple office procedure called an endometrial biopsy.

The Endometrial Biopsy

During an endometrial biopsy, a small plastic cylinder is placed within the cervix. It contains a device that applies mild suction, allowing a portion of endometrial lining to be withdrawn and sent for laboratory analysis. This procedure takes only minutes in the doctor's office, and causes minimal discomfort.

The cellular structure of the endometrium can tell us a great deal as it normally varies in composition throughout the menstrual cycle, as well as when something is awry. (In Chapter Six, we'll discuss the role of the endometrial biopsy in the diagnosis of cancerous and precancerous conditions.) If a woman has anovulatory cycles leading to consecutively missed periods, the endometrium becomes thickly overgrown with tissue—a condition called *endometrial hyperplasia*. This is a proliferative endometrium that has not progressed to the secretory phase in many weeks. The lining has to be rebuilt normally to prevent or stop any abnormal bleeding and to reestablish a normal menstrual pattern.

The "Medical Curettage"

The "standard response" to dysfunctional uterine bleeding is frequently a D&C. This effectively removes the endometrium that may then be studied for abnormalities in the same manner as with the endometrial biopsy. The drawback is that if an underlying hormonal imbalance exists, this cure is short-lived. It only lasts until the next anovulatory cycle causes a recurrence of the problem. Unfortunately, some women have undergone repeated unsuccessful D&Cs only to wind up with a hysterectomy when hormonal therapy would probably have cured their abnormal bleeding without repeated or major surgery!

A medical curettage uses combinations of estrogen and/or progesterone to shed the uterine lining and allow it to begin anew. It is a simple, safe, and inexpensive form of therapy that is successful in about 80 percent of all women. However, it is important to emphasize here that *a medical curettage should only be undertaken after endometrial biopsy definitely rules out any pathology,* specifically cancerous or premalignant lesions.

Specific regimens of estrogen and progesterone vary according to the exact nature of the suspected imbalance and the symptoms a woman may be experiencing. Attention must be paid to individualizing the plan of care for each woman. For example, if a woman has missed her menses and it is suspected that it is because she has failed to produce progesterone, but that her pituitary gland, ovaries, uterus, and estrogen levels are all normal, she can be given a course of progesterone to induce her menses.

However, a woman with severe bleeding requires more complex therapy. We said earlier that missed ovulation causes nonstop estrogen production and accumulation of a hyperplastic endometrium. Once the ovary is no longer capable of maintaining the lining with continued estrogen, it suddenly sloughs, causing profound and unexpected bleeding. Thus it may first be necessary to temporarily replace this estrogen and stop the hemorraging. Afterward, estrogen and progesterone are administered to mimic a normal cycle. Progesterone should convert the proliferative endometrium into a secretory one. Patients need to be carefully monitored over the succeeding months. A repeat endometrial biopsy should be performed to study the appearance of the lining and to insure that things are indeed back to normal.Once these hormones are withdrawn, a normal menstrual period should ensue.

It's worth mentioning here that there have been other medical therapies employed in the treatment of dysfunctional uterine bleeding. They include androgens and androgen derivatives like Danazol, antiprostaglandins and combination progestins such as Norlutate. All of these can play a role in arresting or slowing down menstrual bleeding.

In addition, Clomiphene Citrate, more popularly known as "Clomid," is sometimes used in women with dysfunctional uterine bleeding who desire pregnancy because it is known to induce ovulation. Thus it reverses anovulatory cycles and the abnormal bleeding that accompanies it. However, Clomid therapy must be carefully monitored as it can cause some side effects, including the formation of ovarian cysts.

By far, the most proven remedy for dysfunctional uterine bleeding remains to be estrogen and progesterone—alone or in combination.

Summary

Dysfunctional uterine bleeding is said to be present when all organic causes of abnormal vaginal bleeding have been eliminated. We now know that it is caused by a problem with the secretion of pituitary and/or ovarian hormones. This sometimes interferes with ovulation and always causes an irregular proliferation and shedding of the lining of the uterus. On occasion, dysfunctional uterine bleeding results in missed periods, but it usually causes excessive bleeding at inappropriate times in the cycle.

In Jeffcoate's most recent edition of his work, *Jeffcoate's Principles of Gynaecology*, published in 1987, he advocates hysterectomy as necessary in some cases of dysfunctional uterine bleeding. He says, "In younger women, a radical operation is to be avoided whenever possible but, even in these, there comes a time when hysterectomy with conservation of the ovaries is preferable to incapacity prolonged indefinitely merely for the sake of preserving what is likely to be a very unsatisfactory reproductive function." In my view, it is disheartening to see that Dr. Jeffcoate has not revised his thinking in over 30 years! The many variations of hormonal therapies and the availability of endometrial ablation now makes D&C outmoded and hysterectomy unnecessary.

6

The Spectre of Cancer

Hope and patience are two sovereign remedies for all, the surest reposals, the softest cushions to lean on in adversity.

—*Robert Burton, 1577-1640*

You've seen the scene played on television hundreds of times. The doctor tells the patient, "I'm sorry, Mrs. Jones. You have cancer." The music swells and the drama unfolds. However, we don't imagine that cancer can happen to us. Sadly, cancer strikes in real life thousands of times per year. To be more specific, there were 70,700 cases of female cancer in 1988, resulting in over 23,000 deaths (see Table 6.1).

Perhaps no other word in the English language can so universally conjure up notions of terror in our minds. Immediately, we see certain images. We have certain questions. Can it be cured? Will I be in pain? Am I going to live? Why me?

As we shall see, not all cancers are created equal. Even within the same organ, cancer may have many faces. This presentation is not meant to be a complete and authoritative discussion of gynecological cancer. Rather, it is designed to introduce you to the wide realm of conditions that are cancerous or may be precancerous. It will leave you with a comprehension of the various treatment options, including when hysterectomy may be unavoidable.

We'll begin with a discussion of cervical cancer because it is one of the most common *and* the single most preventable gynecological malignancy.

Table 6.1 Cancer statistics for the United States—What are your chances of developing a pelvic cancer and what are your chances of surviving it? These figures are for the numbers of estimated new cases in the United States for 1990, as well as the five-year survival rates.

Site	New Cases	Survival Rate
Cervix	13,500	67%/88%*
Endometrium	33,000	85%/92%*
Ovary	20,500	38%/85%*
Vagina	<1,000	50%
Vulva	<3,000	80%
Fallopian tubes	<1,000	30%

*The first (and lower) number indicates the overall five-year survival rate. The second (and higher) figure represents the five-year survival rate when the cancer is detected and treated in its earliest stages.

Cancer of the Cervix

What Is Cancer?

Cancer is said to occur when the normal replicating mechanism of the cell becomes subverted and abnormal cells grow and develop uncontrollably. Cells, you will recall, are the building blocks of tissue which in turn makes up the various organs of our bodies. Under the direction of our genetic material, aging cells are constantly being replaced by fresh, new structures. Although we don't completely understand the entire process, our bodies normally regulate the extent and timing of these cellur transformations. When there is irregular growth of abnormal cells and these cells either physically crowd out the normal tissue and/or alter normal cellular functioning, we begin to notice the manifestations of this process as the signs and symptoms of cancer.

Some cancers grow very rapidly; others are slower. This is generally a reflection of their origin. Thus some tissues of the body have a very slow rate of turnover and cancer cells within that tissue will seem to progress at a slower rate. However, because cancer cells lack the inherent protective mechanism of normal cells that tells them when and for how long they should stop reproducing, cancerous cellular growth always overtakes normal cellular growth within that particular organ. For example, even though thyroid tissue and hence thyroid cancer grows very slowly, the cancerous cells quickly crowd out the normal cells. The reason this leads to so much danger and destruction is that cancer cells are unable to correctly carry out the life-sustaining functions of that particular tissue. Yet, they use up the essential nutrients which are then unavailable to the remaining normal structures. Sometimes, they produce chemicals which disrupt the overall physiology of the body. And while they do die, cancer cells reproduce so quickly that their overall numbers are constantly increasing, never decreasing (unless acted on by outside forces). When cancer cells somehow infiltrate the blood, lymph, or surrounding structures, they quickly extend their path of destruction. This is known as *metastasis.*

What Does It Mean If My Pap Smear Is Abnormal?

Cervical cancer is the second most common malignancy of the pelvic organs. One in 63 newborn girls will develop it. In most cases, there are no symptoms, although women may occasionally have some light, irregular vaginal bleeding or a clear, thin discharge. Fortunately, it is a very slow-growing type, and 100 percent curable in the earliest stages. The Pap smear has saved thousands—probably millions—of lives since its development in 1928.

However, it is essential to understand that a Pap test is not infallible—it is merely a *screening test* that allows pathologists to examine exfoliated cells from the cervix and sometimes the uterus. At times, tests will be read as negative because no cancer cells were shed or accumulated on the doctor's spatula when the test was performed. At other times, it may be difficult for a pathologist to pinpoint the exact nature of the problem because the Pap only provides an indirect look at the tissue. Thus anything identified as a potential concern during the performance of this screening test mandates close and complete follow-up by the gynecologist.

Furthermore, because there might have been some irregularity in the technique of obtaining or reading the slides, many gynecologists (myself included) recommend that women have annual Pap smears. The American Cancer Society advocates that Pap smears be performed routinely only every three years once a woman has had two consecutive negative exams. This is because they believe annual Pap smears are not cost-effective and are unnecessary because cervical cancer is such a slowly progressive tumor. For the reasons I've already indicated, I disagree. And, I also want to emphasize that abstaining from Pap smears for three years does not excuse one from a yearly visit to the gynecologist. Annual breast and pelvic exams are crucial to check for other forms of cancer and disease states. It is, therefore, advisable to do a Pap test at the same time.

Finally, it must be remembered that *a Pap smear screens mainly for cervical cancer.* Having annual Pap tests does *not* give us any reliable information about other forms of cancer, such as that of the uterus or ovary. (Cancer cells from these areas may only rarely reveal themselves on a Pap smear if the disease is fairly extensive and the dead cells have migrated into the cervical canal.)

Basically, the cervix is covered with flaky, scaly cells akin to our skin cells known as *squamous epithelium.* Within the os, a different type of epithelial cell is present, known as *columnar epithelium.* The border where these two types of epithelial cells meet is called the *transformation* or *transitional zone.* This is important to know because it is an area frequently associated with either cancerous or precancerous cells.

Beneath this layer of squamous epithelium are the *basal cells.* These are the less mature, rapidly dividing cells that normally should not be present close enough to the surface to be obtained via a Pap smear. Cancerous tissue grows and divides so rapidly that it forces newer or more poorly differentiated cells to within reach of the Pap swab where they will be detected under the microscope by trained pathologists.

Pap smear classifications vary from lab to lab across the country. The most common terminology and their descriptions can be found in Table 6.2.

A negative Pap test will detect what is known as *squamous metaplasia.* Although this might sound ominous, squamous metaplasia indicates completely normal tissue. The next designation is called *atypia* or *inflammation.* This means that some type of irritant or infection is present which has changed the character of the cells, but not in a cancerous fashion. Presumably, the Pap will

Table 6.2 Pap smear classifications—Various terms that may be used by different laboratories in reporting a Pap smear result.

Class I:	Negative (squamous metaplasia)
Class II:	Atypia or inflammation
Class III:	Mild or moderate dysplasia Mild or moderate cervical Intraepithelial neoplasia CIN—Grades I or II
Class IV:	Severe dysplasia Severe cervical intraepithelial neoplasia CIN—Grade III Carcinoma in situ
Class V:	Invasive carcinoma

revert to normal once the cause of the inflammation is discovered and treated. Any designations beyond "atypia" are considered to be precancerous or cancerous conditions. *Dysplasia* or *Cervical Intraepithelial Neoplasia* (CIN) as well as the more advanced *Carcinoma In Situ* are virtually 100 percent curable if caught early.

Cervical Cancer: A Venereal Disease?

In the course of researching cervical cancer, some fascinating associations have been revealed. Demographically speaking, cervical cancer seems to be mostly a disease of the inner city. Although 1 in 63 newborn girls will develop cervical cancer, their risk does not seem to be evenly distributed. Women of lower socioeconomic status are at greatest risk. This is especially true of girls who become sexually active at a young age, who have many partners (especially uncircumcised ones), and many children. One theory to account for this is that the transformation or transitional zone—an area of the cervix particularly susceptible to cancer—is formed during the teen years. Exposure to many partners during adolescence lends itself to exposure to many infectious agents that may then trigger cancer. The herpes virus, and more definitively, the human papilloma viruses (also known as "condyloma" or venereal warts) have been implicated in precancerous changes of the cervix. Other stimuli that have been implicated in cervical cancer include semen and smegma. Among nuns, virgins, and orthodox Jewish women (whose partners are always circumcised), cervical cancer is almost unheard of. Exposure to DES (Diethylstilbestrol) has also been potentially linked to cervical cancer, and more frequent Pap tests are recommended for the women who fall into this category.

The importance of these epidemiologic findings cannot be stressed enough because they mean that cervical cancer is not only detectable (via Pap smear) and curable, but *preventable!*

Colposcopy

The next step in the diagnosis of cervical cancer after a suspicious Pap test is a colposcopic examination. This procedure may be envisioned as an extended speculum exam during which the gynecologist carefully looks at the entire cervix through a magnifying microscopelike device. Often, the cervix may be bathed with a vinegarlike solution to accentuate the architecture of the cells. Biopsies, or small snips of tissue, will be obtained from areas that appear abnormal. In addition, scrapings are obtained from the endocervical canal. This is the channel within the os that is not visible to an examiner. Experts estimate that colposcopy is 95 percent accurate in detecting cervical abnormalities.

The Cure: Laser, Cryosurgery, and Cone Biopsy

When cancer cells of the cervix are "preinvasive" (localized), hysterectomy is *not* necessary. Precancerous changes of the cervix may be obliterated via the laser or by cryosurgery—a freezing procedure that destroys abnormal tissue. There are varying opinions as to whether laser or cryosurgery is preferred for mild dysplasia. Personally, I find that the one drawback to cryosurgery is an inability for the surgeon to control the precise width and depth of penetration. The liquid nitrogen used as the freezing material spreads out in all directions and may even bury the transitional zone more deeply, leading to potential problems in following up on any future lesions. In addition, overzealous cryocautery of the cervix can destroy many of the mucous secreting glands thereby jeopardizing a woman's ability to become pregnant.

When there is a suspicion of more extensive disease, or when colposcopy fails to confirm the findings of several abnormal Pap tests, it is necessary to progress to a more extensive surgical procedure known as a *cone biopsy.*

During conization, a cone-shaped section of tissue is removed from the center of the cervix. These cells are then examined to determine how deeply within the epithelial and/or basal layers the abnormalities exist. While diagnostic, the cone biopsy is also therapeutic. In 85 percent of cases, all of the abnormal tissue is removed and the dysplasia (abnormal growth) will not recur.

Between laser surgery, cryosurgery, and cone biopsy, a vast majority of cervical dysplasias (precancerous tissues) may be obliterated without having to subject women to hysterectomies. However, cone biopsy is not a minor procedure in and of itself. It requires general anesthesia. In addition, 10 to 15 percent of extensive cone biopsies may result in hemorrhagic complications. An overaggressive conization can cause cervical weakness and therefore miscarriage and infertility may ensue.

Is Hysterectomy Ever Necessary for Cervical Cancer?

Unfortunately, the answer to this question is a resounding "yes"! The stages of disease we categorize as cervical cancer fall along a continuum that we may correspond to the Pap smear classifications already described (see Table 6.2). Some cellular changes are considered to be at high risk of progressing to actual cancer, but are still precancerous. These are the mild and moderate dysplasias grouped under CIN Grades I and II or so-called Class III Pap tests. These may be treated with laser or cryosurgery with a fair amount of confidence that any further progression to cancer has been arrested.

Class IV Paps, so-called *carcinoma in situ*, again may permit conservative treatment with local excision usually via cone biopsy. In this case, carcinoma in situ means that there are cancerous cells present, but they have not penetrated deeply into the layers of the cervix nor have they invaded surrounding tissues. Naturally, very careful follow-up is necessary for these women to assure that all cancerous cells were excised and have not recurred. It is also essential to guarantee that the cancerous tissues were genuinely in situ and not invasive.

Truly invasive carcinoma of the cervix (Class V Pap smears) must be treated aggessively. "Real" cancer requires "real" treatment. This means surgery to remove the pelvic organs and nearby lymph nodes to stem the spread of the cancer. While some physicians suggest radiotherapy (destruction of cancerous cells via exposure to strong doses of X rays), it has been my experience that the chance of a successful outcome is greater with surgery. Occasionally, a woman may require radiation therapy prior to surgery in order to shrink extensive tumors so that they are operable. Or, she may have radiotherapy after surgery to erradicate residual disease.

While it must be apparent by now that I *never* resort to hysterectomy when other options are available, with cancer one plays a dangerous game if one tries a "wait and see" approach or attempts a partial measure. In the case of a fibroid, for example, it will not be life-threatening to a woman to attempt to save her precious uterus via a laser ablation or a myomectomy. If such attempts are unsuccessful, one can always resort to hysterectomy as the "final" solution. With cancer, there is no such luxury and there may be no turning back. A woman should *never* hesitate to trade her uterus for her life.

Cancer of the Uterus

Although a woman's uterus is comprised of three distinct layers—the endometrium, the myometrium and the serosa—the vast majority of uterine cancers grow within the endometrium (the innermost layer). Endometrial cancer is the most common of gynecologic cancers. It will strike 1 in 45 newborn girls at some time in their lives, generally when they approach menopause. Like cervical cancer, not all of these 45 hypothetical newborns have an equal risk. Unlike cervical cancer, endometrial cancer is demographically linked to the suburbs. In addition, genetic and environmental factors may play a role, since there seems to be a tendency for this type of cancer to develop in certain families, especially among Jewish women and among women who eat high fat, high cholesterol diets. There have also been associations made between endometrial cancer and obesity, diabetes, and high blood pressure.

But the brightest warning lights flash when a woman suffers from hormonal imbalances of the type we discussed in Chapter Five. Abnormal ovulation, prolonged estrogen stimulation, and dysfunctional uterine bleeding are all linked to endometrial cancer. Indeed, they may be precursors in some women.

Hyperplasia

As explained in Chapter Five, a woman may miss several consecutive menstrual periods due to hormonal abnormalities that fail to trigger the normal sequence of events leading up to menstruation, including ovulation and surges of estrogen and progesterone. When this happens, the endometrial lining thickens, becoming more and more crowded with glands. This condition is known as hyperplasia. Initially, these glands grow in abnormal numbers, however, they maintain their normal structure and configuration. However, left unchecked, these glands possess the ability to grow in abnormal form and progress to cancer.

Any woman with abnormal uterine bleeding, including irregular menses, needs to have an endometrial biopsy. (Remember: Pap smears do *not* screen for endometrial cancer.) Normally, the biopsy will show either a secretory or proliferative lining, depending on what phase of the menstrual cycle she is in. If, however, the endometrium is hyperplastic, treatment must be initiated.

Like cervical cancer, endometrial hyperplasia is a continuum. Cystic and adenomatous hyperplasia are terms for tissue that is still comprised of normal cells, but at increasingly high risk of progressing to endometrial cancer. Cystic hyperplasia is really of no consequence. However, anywhere from 15 to 30 percent of women with adenomatous hyperplasia will develop endometrial cancer in three to five years. With "atypical" adenomatous hyperplasia, there is already some abnormal cell and glandular formation, thus cancer is but a step away.

Treatment: Hyperplasia and Beyond

When hormonal imbalances and endometrial abnormalities are detected early enough, they may be reversed rather simply by treatments with potent progesterones. Portions of the lining are initially removed during the endometrial biopsy and then progesterone accomplishes a medical curettage (see Chapter Five) to slough the remaining abnormal tissue. After several cycles of progesterone, the body often resumes its normal functioning and the endometrium reverts to normal.

However, the treatment of adenomatous hyperplasia in this manner must be approached as a calculated risk. Frequent endometrial biopsies are required to assure that there is no recurrence. Abnormal tissue missed on biopsy may mean that the disease may progress to a more serious stage before it is detected and thus require more aggressive therapy than if it were caught earlier. Atypical adenomatous hyperplasia is particularly pernicious, therefore, a maximum of three to six months of medical therapy with strong progesterones is all that should be attempted. If there is no resolution of the hyperplasia within this time, then hysterectomy is recommended.

Again, as with cervical cancer, cancer of the endometrium requires hysterectomy. Depending on the stage of the disease, the uterus alone may be removed or more radical surgery involving the removal of other pelvic organs and lymph nodes may be required. Radiation therapy may also be performed for extensive cases. In some centers, radiation therapy in conjunction with surgery is used routinely.

Estrogen and Endometrial Cancer

Years ago, the earliest forms of birth control pills contained very high doses of estrogen, sometimes without any progesterone present to "oppose" it. Studies showed that women who took these pills were at increased risk of developing endometrial cancer, and these pills were taken off the market over a decade ago. Some women still have lingering fears about taking hormones, either as oral contraceptives or to reduce the adverse effects of menopause. Recent studies seem to show that hormonal regimens that contain both estrogen *and* progesterone do *not* place a woman at higher risk for uterine cancer *and* may even *lower* her risk. (More about this will be discussed in Chapter 9.)

Are You at Risk for Endometrial or Cervical Cancer?

Endometrial and cervical cancer are the two most common types of malignancies afflicting women. Yet, the characteristics of the women who develop them are dramatically different. The following list allows you to compare and contrast the risk factors for each.

You may be at risk for cervical cancer if you . . .

- Began having intercourse as a teenager.

- Have or had many sexual partners. (*Note:* This also applies if you have been monogamous, but *your partner* has or had multiple sexual contacts.)

- Have contracted certain sexually transmitted diseases, especially genital warts (condyloma accumunata) or genital herpes (herpes simplex, type II.)

- Have a partner who has not been circumcised.

- Have a partner who has contracted penile cancer.

- Have been exposed to DES.

You may lower your risk of contracting cervical cancer if you . . .

- Practice "safe sex." In other words, have open and honest discussions with your partner(s) concerning your sexual histories. Get to know the men you are dating, and with whom you are planning intimacy. Use barrier methods of contraception, such as condoms and diaphragms, as these prevent the transmission of venereal diseases.

- Examine yourself (and your partner(s)) for any sores, growths or discharges in the genital area that may signal a sexually transmitted disease. Seek medical attention promptly if you discover something that concerns you.

- Have annual pelvic exams and Pap tests. Follow your doctor's advice for more frequent exams if you have been exposed to DES or have had an abnormal Pap in the past.

- Practice good hygiene and a healthy lifestyle. For example, women who smoke or eat poorly are at a greater risk of developing any kind of cancer.

You may be at risk for developing endometrial cancer if you . . .

- Are overweight.

- Have diabetes or high blood pressure.

- Have had problems with ovulation and dysfunctional uterine bleeding.

- Experienced menopause after the age of 50.

- Have a family history of endometrial cancer.

- Eat a high fat, high cholesterol diet.

You may lower your risk of developing endometrial cancer if you:

- Eat sensibly to reduce your weight and dietary intake of fats and cholesterol. Increasing your fiber may also be helpful.

- Make good health a priority, by seeing your physician and following his advice to maintain blood pressure or diabetes under control.

- Have annual pelvic and Pap smears and report any abnormal vaginal bleeding at once.

Uterine Sarcomas

Ninety-five to 99 percent of uterine cancers are of the endometrium. However, for completeness' sake, it's necessary to briefly discuss sarcomas. These are rare malignancies that arise in the muscle or connective tissue of the uterus. (We've already mentioned leiomyosarcomas in Chapter Three.) The prognosis for this type of cancer, like endometrial cancer, is good *but only* if caught in the earliest stages. Treatment options include pelvic surgery with or without radiation and/or chemotherapy.

Cancer of the Ovary

Naturally, when a U.S. president or a show business celebrity develops a form of cancer, it is brought to the forefront of public attention through intense media exposure. Suddenly, where we may never have even heard of a disease, now we know its signs and symptoms, its cure rate, and the medical tests we may have been neglecting that may alert us to its presence in our bodies. Never is such an occurence as poignant and frightening as when cancer strikes someone young, vibrant, attractive and likable: someone like ourselves. The death of Gilda Radner, a talented comedienne in her forties made many women acutely aware of their own risk of ovarian cancer. Ovarian cancer is a very serious disease when it strikes. Fortunately, it is relatively rare, afflicting just over 1 out of every 70 women in their lifetimes. A variety of surprising characteristics have been linked to an increased risk of developing ovarian cancer ranging from having Type A blood to being resistant to mumps! But a particularly disturbing statistic reveals that women with breast cancer are twice as likely to also develop ovarian cancer and vice versa.

Despite its relative rarity, ovarian cancer is the leading cause of gynecologic cancer-related deaths. Eleven thousand lives are lost to this dreaded tumor every year. Even more tragic is the fact that the incidence seems to have risen in the past generation with no progress having been made in early detection and cure.

"Silent but Deadly"

Ovarian cancer has been called "silent but deadly." It's silent because its vague symptoms of abdominal discomfort, bloating, and other mild digestive disturbances might be confused with an entire litany of other medical conditions from heartburn to gallbladder disease. And it's deadly because the ovary is a very complex organ with a variety of tissue types—all of which have the potential to comprise the "family" of malignancies we know as ovarian cancer. All progress relatively rapidly and none seem to respond well to the therapies we currently have available. The combined equation of a cancer that does not generally identify itself until its advanced stages and one that is poorly responsive to treatment add up to the silent but deadly characterization.

Yet, no matter how bleak the picture of ovarian cancer seems, it is *not* a universal death sentence. In my practice, I have been very fortunate to have seen very few cases of gynecologic cancers of any type. Francine is one of my few patients with ovarian cancer. She first came to me 14 years ago. Francine is the shining example of never giving up hope despite the odds:

> *In 1975, when Francine was 42 years old, she developed pain on her right side which was accompanied by nausea and bloating. She could no longer tolerate the rich foods she had often liked to eat in the past. Initially, her internist diagnosed gallbladder disease. But when tests for this condition were negative, Francine was referred to me for further evaluation.*
>
> *A pelvic exam revealed a suspicious mass on the right side which was confirmed on ultrasound. On subsequent surgery, Francine was found to have endometriosis in her right ovary with cancerous tumors in her left ovary. She underwent extensive surgery involving the removal of her uterus, ovaries, fallopian tubes, and portions of her omentum. This was followed by a two-year course of chemotherapy.*
>
> *Now, at age 56, Francine is a vibrant and active person. She shows absolutely no signs or symptoms of a recurrence of the ovarian cancer. And while she endured a hellish two years, Francine may now be considered to be cured of her disease.*

Diagnosis and Treatment

As we mentioned earlier, ovarian cancer is difficult to detect. The symptoms are nebulous and the ovary relatively inaccessible to routine examination. An ovary with a malignant tumor already brewing may still be too small to be evident on bimanual examination. Pap smears, biopsies, and so forth are not applicable as screening tools here for obvious reasons. Even CAT scans may not be helpful in early diagnosis, although investigations into the use of MRI are progressing. There are some blood tests, including those that monitor liver enzymes, hormone levels, and tumor markers (like serum Calcium 125) that offer information regarding the progress of the disease. However, they are not reliable *screening tests* for the presence of ovarian cancer in their present stage of development.

Some doctors now recommend screening vaginal ultrasound examinations for women at high risk for ovarian cancer, including women in their late reproductive and menopausal years. Women who appear to have significant ovarian cysts on sonogram and women who have any cancer symptoms, such as they are, should have frequent ultrasound examinations. Although imperfect, at least this technique offers some chance at early detection. And, any woman over 40 with an ovarian cyst that does not resolve in a few menstrual cycles must have an exploratory laparoscopy or laparotomy. The extent of the surgery depends on the size, the nature, and the degree of suspicion a particular ovarian tumor possesses.

As one might imagine, the treatment of ovarian cancer should be as aggressive as the disease. It frequently involves removal of the pelvic organs along with the appendix and portions of the intestinal covering known as the *omentum*. In addition, radiation and chemotherapy are often employed as adjuncts to surgery.

Cancer of the Fallopian Tubes

Cancer of the fallopian tubes is one of the rarest of all cancers. In fact, most gynecologists will never see a case during their entire careers. It afflicts 1 of every 1,000 women, but, because of its rarity, no epidemiologic statistics exist to identify women who may be at higher risk for developing it. While it has been suggested that chronic inflammation of the fallopian tubes may be a precursor, this is difficult to pin down, since there are so many cases of salpingitis (inflammation of the oviducts) as compared to so few cases of cancer.

Although there is a myriad of symptoms that may be associated with this type of malignancy, none is characteristic or dramatic enough to raise the red flag. For example, a woman might have vaginal bleeding, pain, or discharge. She may feel a sense of pressure or bloating in her abdomen. A mass may be felt during a pelvic examination. All of these may be symptoms of other, more common forms of cancer *or* other noncancerous conditions, such as pelvic inflammatory disease or ectopic pregnancy.

The treatment and prognosis of fallopian tube cancer unfortunately follow along the same lines as ovarian cancer. Difficult to detect in its earliest stages, this cancer is rapidly progressive and destructive. Surgery and radiation are utilized to attempt to eradicate the malignant tissue.

Cancer of the Vulva and Vagina

We began this discussion with a cancer that is frequently preventable and curable and we can end this way as well. Cancers of the vulva, like cervical cancers, seem to have links to the herpes and human papilloma viruses. Poor hygiene practices may allow these infectious, potentially precancerous irritants to remain on the surface of these structures, thus opening the door to cancer. However,

---

Cancer: A Self-Help Guide
A Checklist of Pelvic Cancer's Major Signs and Symptoms

See your doctor if you notice any of the following . . .

- Any unusual growths or sores on or near your vulva.

  * The genital warts (condyloma; HPV) that seem to be linked to cervical cancer look like flesh-tone cauliflower-like pimples that may appear singly or in clusters. They are painless.

  ** Herpes simplex, also a possible precursor of cervical cancer, generally appears as a painful or itchy shallow ulcer or blister that may contain a yellow fluid. They may appear singly or in clusters.

  *** Vulvar cancers appear as raised sores or ulcers that are painful, may ooze or bleed, and don't heal.

- Vaginal discharge.

- Abnormal uterine bleeding. Any change in the normal flow, that is a change in the amount, duration, consistency, or timing of vaginal bleeding.

- Pelvic pain.

- Spotting after intercourse.

- Palpable lumps in your abdomen or a noticeable bloating or increase in abdominal girth.

- Abdominal pain, nausea, vomiting, gas, constipation, weight loss, or loss of appetite.

- Swollen glands in the groin area.

- Painful, frequent, or difficult urination.

unlike cervical cancer, these malignancies are very rare (only slightly more common than fallopian tube cancer) and almost always strike women in their late sixties and early seventies.

Finally, we have vaginal cancer. Only five women in one million develop vaginal carcinoma and, as with vulvar cancer, these women are well past menopause. The significant exception to this rule are the daughters of women who took DES (Diethylstilbestrol) during their pregnancies to avert miscarriages. These DES daughters develop vaginal cancers early in life. (The peak incidence seems to be at about age 19, with about 1 out of every 1,000 women exposed affected.)

Although cancers of the vulva and vagina are rare, easily detectable, and highly curable in the earliest stages, a criminal number of women die from them every year. This can only be attributed to ignorance and negligence. Older women and their doctors may omit Pap smears and pelvic exams believing them to be unnecessary, uncomfortable, and embarrassing when a woman is "so old," is no longer sexually active, or may have even had a hysterectomy. They forget that these women are in the highest risk group.

Both vulvar and vaginal cancers are susceptible to a variety of treatment options falling short of hysterectomy. They include: laser surgery, cryosurgery, and treatment with radiation or topical chemotherapeutic agents.

Summary

Thousands of hysterectomies are performed in the United States every year for gynecologic cancer. Most are justified. Unfortunately, once a flagrant malignancy has developed, nothing short of its total obliteration may be attempted at the risk of a woman's life. However, I'd like the emphasis here to be on the positive, not on the negative—on the potential for prevention and minimizing one's risk of developing a cancer in the first place.

We've seen that certain cancers, such as those of the cervix, vulva, and vagina are linked to certain diseases and irritants. Women can avoid these by taking certain commonsense precautions. These include: practicing good hygiene, using condoms, and keeping their Pap smears up-to-date. Other cancers seem to be more common among women who are obese, since fat stores estrogen. These so-called estrogen dependent cancers include cancer of the breast, ovary, and endometrium. It is, therefore, no surprise that eating a diet low in fat and cholesterol as well as high in fiber will decrease a woman's risk of developing ovarian and endometrial carcinomas.

But even after decades of research, so much about cancer—its causes and cures—remains a mystery. Sadly, as we continue to pollute our environment and expose ourselves to so many potential carcinogens in our air, water, food, homes, and workplaces, cancer rates mount. It is difficult to say what is ultimately responsible for these frightening statistics. Perhaps it is these environmental factors, or perhaps it is the mere fact that a century ago women died of infectious diseases or childbirth long before their cells aged enough to mutate into cancer. Most likely, it is a combination of many factors including genetic composition as well as exposure to toxins.

While there may be some risk factors each of us has which we cannot change, we can all make an impact on many other risks. Currently women have the edge over men when it comes to cancer deaths. This may be because they smoke less (although this is changing), they drink less, they seek medical care on a more regular basis, and they have less occupational exposure. Let's hope that women do not fall behind in the battle against cancer. A healthy lifestyle which includes a nurtritious diet, a minimum of stress, sound medical care, and a safe environment will keep women's immune systems in top fighting shape to do battle against the cancer foe . . . and to win.

7

Prolapse, Pelvic Inflammatory Disease, and Pregnancy

The whole uterus is protruded from its seat and lodged between the woman's thighs—an incredible affliction. . . . It takes place from abortion, great concussions, and laborious parturition. . . . If it does not prove fatal, the woman lives for a long time, seeing parts that ought not be seen, and nursing externally and fondling the womb. . . . Sometimes the mouth of the womb only, as far as its neck, protrudes, and retreats inwardly if the uterus be made to smell a fetid fumigation, and the woman also attracts it in if she herself smells fragrant odors. But by the hands of the midwife it readily returns inward when gently pressed, if anointed beforehand with the emolient plaster. . . .
—*Aretaeus the Cappadocian, A.D. 81–138.*

Up to 1984, the most recent year for which nationwide hysterectomy statistics are available, prolapse of the uterus accounted for 21 percent of all hysterectomies performed. Another 21 percent of these operations were performed for various miscellaneous conditions (not including fibroids, endometriosis, and cancer)—the most significant of which were pelvic infections or conditions related to pregnancy. Clearly, then, this book would not be complete without a discussion of these potential causes of hysterectomy. I say "potential causes" because *none of them necessarily need to result in hysterectomy.*

Prolapse: Hernias of the Pelvic Floor

Prolapse is the term used to describe what happens when weakened support structures allow the uterus to descend from the pelvic cavity into the vagina or the vagina itself to turn inward and drop toward the vulva. When the uterus prolapses, it drags with it the upper portions of the vagina and in rare, severe cases, the entire cervix and uterus protrude entirely outside the body.

Prolapse has been recognized from earliest times, and it's interesting and amusing to read how our physician predecessors accounted for this condition. For example, both the ancient Egyptians and the ancient Greeks believed that the uterus had a personality all its own, and therefore could move about independently and at will. Thus, if it were attracted to something outside of the body, the uterus might migrate toward it. Here, a second century A.D. Greek physician, Aretaeus the Cappadocian, writes:

> In the middle of the flanks of women lies the womb, a female viscus, closely resembling an animal, for it moved of itself hither and thither in the flanks, also upwards in a direct line below the cartilage of the thorax, and also obliquely to the right of the left, either to the liver or the spleen; and it likewise is subjected to prolapse downwards, and in a word is altogether erratic. It delights also in fragrant smells and advances toward them, and it has an aversion to fetid smells and flees from them; and on the whole the womb is like an animal within an animal.

Centuries later, the Victorian Age brought yet another "explanation." Prolapse, it was believed, came about when a woman engaged in activities she really wasn't designed for, like singing, dancing, horseback riding, skating, wearing dresses with tight lacings, and worst of all—masturbation! Truthfully, Aretaeus was probably more on target when he blamed strenuous labor as a cause back in early Christian times. Certainly Victorian women were more at risk of developing a prolapsed uterus from the obstetrical practices of the time as well as from their physical labors than from singing or skating.

Still, uterine prolapse through the ages has been a common affliction, especially for older women. Although overall prolapse-related hysterectomy statistics are about 21 percent, this figure doubles to 41 percent in women over age 65. In other words, 4 out of every 10 women undergoing hysterectomy after their sixty-fifth birthday do so for uterine prolapse. But is hysterectomy always necessary?

Twenty-five years ago, we often used mild prolapse of the uterus to justify a hysterectomy to a hospital commitee that would otherwise have required a woman to have as many as six children before she could be sterilized. We'd place an instrument on her cervix, and attempt to pull it down into the vagina so as to be able to say that she had a so-called uterine prolapse with traction. Fortunately, these tactics are considered to be unnecessary and unethical today, when no woman should have a hysterectomy suggested to her solely for sterilization purposes. (Although unfortunately, some of these practices still continue!) In actual fact, very few women—even those who do have legitimate prolapse—require hysterectomy today.

What Happens

Think of a prolapse as a hernia or bulging of tissue that occurs within the vagina. The uterus, vagina, bladder, and rectum are all held in place by a unified system of supporting ligaments, muscles, and other tissues that resemble a sling. When a weakness develops in these structures, there will be a sagging of this sling that then causes a protrusion into the usually taut vaginal wall.

Normally, only a small portion of the neck of the uterus (the cervix) is present at the very top of the vagina. As we've already briefly mentioned, if its support structures loosen, this organ will then drop down further into the vagina by virtue of its weight and the pull of gravity. (See Figure 7.1.) The uterus cannot prolapse without carrying along with it portions of the vagina and thus causing a "vaginal prolapse." (When the uterus falls, it literally turns the vaginal wall "inside out.") On the contrary, the vagina can prolapse independent of the uterus and in doing so, can affect a woman's bladder or bowel functions.

When a weakness in the vagina occurs in its upper portion, the bladder, which lies directly above it, may lose its "footing," and drop down so that it is bulging into the vagina. This condition is called a *cystocele*. (If only the *urethra*, or tube through which the urine actually exits the body is involved, this is known as a *urethrocele*.)

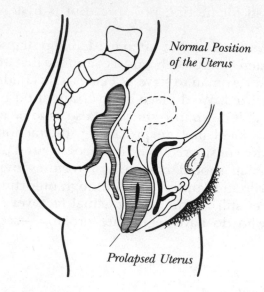

Normal Position
of the Uterus

Prolapsed Uterus

Figure 7.1   Uterine prolapse—The uterus drops down into the vagina due to weakening of its support structure.

If, however, the weakness develops in the lower wall of the vagina, loops of intestines (an *enterocele*) or the rectum itself may protrude into the vaginal walls, resulting in a *rectocele*.

Why It Happens

It's not entirely clear what the direct cause of these conditions is, although certain factors are known to increase the likelihood of developing a prolapse. Perhaps the most frequently implicated of these are pregnancy and childbirth. But let's look more closely at these so-called predisposing factors.

Interestingly, when women with known uterine prolapse become pregnant, it is usually only in the earliest stages of pregnancy that their condition is aggravated. Once the womb enlarges, it rests on the pelvic brim and is kept from descending further into the vagina. Therefore, pregnancy probably does not cause or exacerbate a uterine prolapse, contrary to popular belief.

Labor is another situation entirely. A prolapsed uterus is rarely seen in women who have only delivered via cesarean section. But what is puzzling about this alleged cause is the observation that some women can endure multiple or extremely traumatic births without ever developing a prolapse while other women need never have a child to develop one. Clearly, then, other factors are involved.

Because there seems to be a strong family history associated with this condition, it may be that some women are naturally prone to develop a prolapse due to an inherent weakness of the muscles and tissues that support the uterus and vagina. For these women, it is particularly important to have expert obstetrical care to avoid events that might trigger a prolapse in those who are so susceptible. For example, while women these days are anxious to avoid episiotomies (a small surgical incision that is made in the perineum to enlarge the vaginal opening so that it may accommodate the baby's head), they may be inviting prolapse at a later date by sustaining vaginal tears and other injuries from excessive and prolonged efforts at delivery. Thus the desire to avoid an episiotomy must be balanced by the desire to avoid future prolapse. Furthermore, you can help to minimize the risk of childbirth-related prolapse by doing Kegel exercises (see the section on Kegel exercises in this chapter) and avoiding constipation during and after your pregnancy.

It's important to realize that women can, but usually do not develop prolapse immediately after their labor and deliveries. It is perhaps during that period of time when the weakness first develops. However, it is generally years later, once a woman undergoes menopause and its associated changes in the genitalia, that the actual prolapse occurs.

Ironically, *hysterectomy may be both the cause and the cure of a vaginal prolapse!* In some cases, the surgical removal of the uterus, especially when it is performed via the vaginal route (see Chapter 9), can cause a weakness in the vagina resulting in prolapse. If the surgeon is not careful in his technique, a woman may need *another operation* to repair and strengthen the vagina posthysterectomy.

When Do You Need Hysterectomy?

As a general rule, hysterectomy can be *avoided* in most cases of uterine, vaginal, bladder, and rectal prolapses. In the majority of cases, it really depends on the severity of the prolapse and how uncomfortable a woman becomes as a result. In other words, because a prolapse is *never* a life-threatening condition, and *very rarely* causes even a serious problem, the best advice is: "don't bother it if it doesn't bother you." The next question is, how might it bother you?

Naturally, the symptoms depend on the structures involved. Slight uterine prolapse are rarely noticeable. As the uterus protrudes further, a woman might feel a sensation of heaviness, dragging or fullness in her vagina or lower abdomen. Medical intervention (but *not* hysterectomy) is only necessary when the cervix and/or uterus actually protrude from the vulva because they may develop infected sores from the irritation of being exposed to the outside.

Cystoceles have the potential to pose more problems, although they don't necessarily do so. Many women function perfectly well with cystoceles they are unaware of. However, cystoceles are frequently blamed for a condition called *stress incontinence.* This is a condition where sudden movements that exert pressure on the perineal area, like laughing, coughing, or sneezing, cause women to leak small amounts of urine. In actual fact, researchers find stress incontinence to be *as common in women without prolapse as in women with prolapse!* Furthermore, the surgery involved in *correcting* uterine prolapse may actually *contribute* to stress incontinence and, at best, may not correct it.

More specifically, because a woman has a uterine prolapse or a cystocele doesn't automatically mean that she has lost control of her bladder function as a result. A cystocele is purely an *anatomical defect* that is sometimes completely symptom-free. In these situations, *correcting a cystocele may actually cause a stress incontinence after surgery that was not there before surgery* because it can alter the inherent angle of the bladder! You *do not need* and *should not have* surgery to correct an asymptomatic cystocele unless you're looking for trouble.

Supposing, however, that you do have a prolapse and some stress incontinence. Then, you may need surgery. However, first a series of tests called *urodynamics* (bladder muscle tone studies) need to be performed by a urologist to assure that the incontinence is not from a neurological problem or other physiologic cause requiring *medical* not surgical intervention.

Thus women should be very skeptical of surgery meant to reverse stress incontinence, and certainly need to undergo thorough testing for other, underlying urinary conditions before consenting to it lest they be bitterly disappointed with the results.

Besides stress incontinence, cystoceles may rarely cause other conditions that necessitate surgical repair (but not necessarily hysterectomy). The bladder is shaped somewhat like a horizontal balloon with a "neck" at its base ending in the urethra. (See Figure 7.2.) Sometimes with a cystocele, the balloon portion of the bladder drops down lower than the neck thus impeding the flow of urine. A woman may have difficulty emptying her bladder. As a result, she may constantly feel the urge to urinate, but may only be able to eliminate small amounts. Eventually, as urine accumulates in the bladder, she may develop frequent infections causing painful urination.

There are various approaches to repairing a cystocele, including lifting the bladder from above through an incision in the abdomen or opening the vaginal wall and pushing up the bladder from below. In either case, as with stress incontinence, it's imperative that whatever symptoms a woman is experiencing should be attributed solely to a defect in her anatomy and *not* from any problem in the functioning of her bladder itself. Again, if the latter is the case, cystocele repairs will be useless, and may even make matters worse. Unfortunately, even under the best circumstances, cystocele repairs are not a guaranteed cure, since the weakness of the tissues can return. Thus, before considering surgery for a cystocele causing stress incontinence, a woman should try to alleviate her systems by strengthening her tissues with exercises and/or estrogen replacement therapy.

Hysterectomy need only accompany cystocele repair when the uterus itself is also significantly prolapsed. If this is not the case, adding hysterectomy to cystocele repair only makes the surgery and its aftermath more complicated. Unfortunately, in many cases, the supporting tissues that have become so weak as to allow bulging of the bladder into the vagina have also caused a dropping down of the uterus. And, permanently repairing a prolapse of the uterus requires its removal. This is because the uterus acts like a piston which pushes down in response to abdominal pressure. Thus, as long as it is present, the uterus has the potential to prolapse again, thus necessitating repeated surgery.

A rectocele, again, is usually asymptomatic and little cause for concern. While women with rectoceles may complain of backaches,

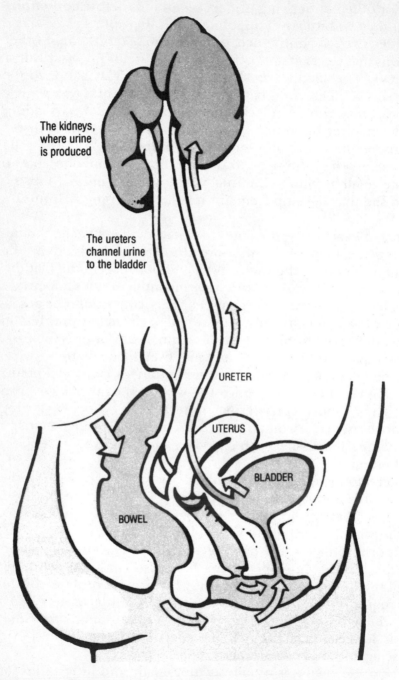

The kidneys, where urine is produced

The ureters channel urine to the bladder

URETER

UTERUS

BLADDER

BOWEL

Figure 7.2   The female urinary tract, side view.

Prolapse: A Self-Help Guide

Symptoms to Look For . . .

- A fleshy protrusion that is palpable inside the vagina or visible outside the vagina, especially when you strain, cough, or laugh.

- A sensation of fullness, heaviness, or pressure within the vagina or lower abdomen.

- Frequent bladder infections, with its associated burning pain, urge to urinate, more frequent urination, urinary retention, and/or blood-tinged urine.

- Leakage of urine or feces with sneezing, coughing, laughing, or straining (stress incontinence).

- Bowel movement disturbances, such as difficulty in moving your bowels or completely emptying your rectum.

- Lower back pain.

there is usually another underlying cause of the back pain unrelated to the rectocele. The main problem with a rectocele may be difficulty in moving one's bowels and completely emptying the rectum. Interestingly, a previously "silent" rectocele may suddenly become troublesome once the uterus is removed, so hysterectomy should never be suggested for this reason. If hysterectomy is necessary for another cause, it's important that any large rectoceles also be eliminated at the same time.

Operations, called vaginal repairs, done to correct cystoceles, rectoceles, and vaginal prolapses frequently cause more problems than they cure. As mentioned earlier, they may cause or worsen stress incontinence. In addition, they may lead to sexual difficulties, particularly from a surgically narrowed or shortened vagina. Furthermore, we already know the multitude of problems that hysterectomy can cause. Most are not worth risking for the relatively simple and benign condition of a prolapsed uterus, unless it is truly hindering the quality of a woman's life. Furthermore, there are other alternatives that do not involve surgery.

For example, you might be able to avoid needing a surgical repair of a cystocele (if it is not as yet causing complications) by performing the exercises explained in the subsequent section.

Self-Help and Nonsurgical Treatments

Kegel Exercises

A California physician named Dr. Arnold Kegel developed these exercises to help women to strengthen the muscles of their pelvic floor. While they are fairly simple to learn and can be performed virtually anywhere, like any exercise, they require persistence and perseverence to obtain successful results. A stronger pelvic floor not only might improve the symptoms of prolapse and stress incontinence, but also frequently enhances sexual pleasure and helps younger women to prepare for childbirth. Here's how they are done.

To begin, a woman must locate exactly which muscle group she needs to work on. To locate the correct muscles, try to stop and start your stream of urine, or, alternately, attempt to squeeze your partner's penis during intercourse. Once you've determined the correct muscle group, you're ready to start your exercise regimen.

Contract, or tighten, these muscles for two or three seconds and then relax them in an alternating pattern of contraction and release for a cycle of 10 repetitions. You can gradually increase the number of cycles you perform each day until you are doing 20 groups of 10 Kegel exercises. This may take a month or two to work up to.

Remember that you can do these exercises while you are otherwise engaged, whether you are standing on line in the bank or sitting at your desk in the office.

Pessaries

If a woman is unwilling or unable to undergo a surgical repair of a uterine prolapse, a pessary may be the answer. This is a devise made of plastic or rubber that fits firmly in the vagina and physically supports the uterus. They come in a variety of models, including those that are inserted into the vagina and then inflated with a small air pump as well as those that are of a fixed size and shape. A pessary does not cure prolapse; it merely holds up the tissues. It may be inconvenient for an active woman or one who frequently engages in intercourse. Likewise, the woman in poor health may find it cumbersome to insert or uncomfortable to wear. However, it is certainly a simple solution, free of the complications of surgery. For Millie, it was the answer to her prayers.

Millie is a vegetable farmer who is on her feet many hours of the day, despite her age of 62. She leads an active life, which includes not only physical labor, but attending to her husband and six grandchildren. Yet, she does not desire surgery for her uterine prolapse. Instead, she uses her pessary to avert the discomforts of her prolapsed uterus whenever necessary, inserting it and removing it at her convenience, such as when she desires intercourse.

As with women who prefer the convenience of pills or IUDs over diaphragms, not every woman may elect to use a pessary. If a woman has significant symptoms from vaginal or uterine prolapse, and she prefers the surgical solution over exercises or the need to deal with a pessary, that is perfectly acceptable. The key here is that the choice is *hers and not her physician's.*

Pelvic Inflammatory Disease

Pelvic Inflammatory Disease (PID) is the term used to describe a massive infection that involves the cervix (*cervicitis*), uterus (*endometritis*), fallopian tubes (*salpingitis*) and/or ovaries (*oophoritis*). Prior to the advent of antibiotics, women frequently died from PID because it progressed to the point that their fallopian tubes swelled with pus until they literally resembled sausages. Rupture of these tubal and/or ovarian abscesses led to sepsis and subsequent death. Today, the disease rarely progresses to this extent and is a very infrequent cause of hysterectomy.

Although other means may occasionally result in pelvic infection (e.g., the introduction of bacteria during an abortion procedure or an IUD insertion), PID is considered for all intents and purposes to be a sexually transmitted disease. It most commonly occurs when the microorganisms causing gonorrhea or chlamydia enter the vagina and ascend into the pelvic cavity. Sometimes a woman may find herself quite ill, with such symptoms as: vaginal discharge, abnormal bleeding, abdominal pain, fever, chills, nausea, vomiting, painful urination, or discomfort during intercourse. Unfortunately, at other times, a lowgrade PID (particularly from chlamydia) may linger with vague or absent symptoms until there is massive damage, most frequently including permanent scarring of the fallopian tubes resulting in infertility or ectopic pregnancy. Or, a woman may suffer with prolonged pelvic pain that has not been properly identified as a chronic or recurrent PID. The medically indigent often suffer recurring infection and escape diagnosis. These women do not receive the essential antibiotics they need at the first hint of a problem. This limited access to medical treatment results in a more advanced state of pelvic destruction.

Left untreated, PID can cause complications extending beyond even infertility. Pockets of infected material, called abscesses, may form in the tubes or ovaries. Furthermore, the infection may spread into the abdominal cavity where there may be damage to the liver and intestines. Although rare, these complications are life-threatening.

While there is no reason why the spread of PID cannot be stemmed long before it reaches these very serious stages, this is the only case where hysterectomy may still occasionally need to be performed—*as a last resort*. First, a woman may need to be hospitalized and placed on strong doses of intravenous antibiotics. If this is ineffective, the next step is to perform an operative laparoscopy, during which the infected fallopian tubes can be drained of their purulent material, repaired, or even removed when absolutely necessary.

The key to avoiding hysterectomy with PID is early, aggressive, and thorough treatment with antibiotics and surgical techniques that stop short of having to remove the uterus. In this manner, women can avoid chronic, resistent infections involving massive areas of the pelvis and bowels that are literally irreversible by any other means.

Pregnancy

In 1869, Dr. Horatio Storer performed the first so-called "cesarean hysterectomy." In those days, according to experts of the time, mothers requiring cesarean sections might die as frequently as 95 percent of the time, compared with only a 5 percent mortality rate when the uterus was removed along with the baby.

Today, of course, dramatically different statistics apply. Only about 1 percent of all pregnancies result in hysterectomy. Some of these are elective, because the mother wishes sterilization (*this is ill-advised*) or has another gynecological condition that the surgeon feels calls for hysterectomy. (Again, this is ill-advised because pregnant women are much more likely to hemorrhage during pelvic surgery as a result of their increased blood supply.)

The remaining causes of obstetrical hysterectomy are generally justified, but are fortunately *very rare*. In fact, I can recall only one case in my practice when a woman, who had had many children, actually developed a tear in her uterus (ruptured uterus) while giving birth. This was accompanied by massive bleeding. The only recourse in this case was hysterectomy to save her life.

In very rare instances, and usually when women have large, vertical incisions, the uterus may rupture at the site of a previous cesarean section scar when women attempt to deliver vaginally in a subsequent pregnancy. Rupture is sometimes associated with severe bleeding which may not be compensated for by transfusions, and thus necessitates emergency hysterectomy. However, for the most part, a ruptured uterus can be repaired and thus women can usually be spared hysterectomy.

Aside from a ruptured uterus, uncontrollable hemorrhage occasionally happens when the placenta is in an abnormal position, or fails to separate from the uterus properly after delivery of the baby. Sometimes, a woman might have a blood clotting problem that arises at the time of delivery secondary to an obstetrical complication where amniotic fluid enters her bloodstream. Again, this is a rare occurence. In these cases, if more conservative measures, such as blood transfusion or a tying off of the hypogostic vessels (the main blood supply to the uterus) involved fail to stem the hemorrhage, hysterectomy is unavoidable.

While this is certainly a tragedy when it happens to a young woman, there can be no wavering when an obstetrical catastrophe forces a doctor to remove the uterus to save the mother's life. Usually, the cervix and the ovaries are preserved in the interest of performing a safe and speedy operation because the mother's life is in jeopardy.

Summary

A variety of miscellaneous, rare and/or benign conditions were the cause of approximately 40 percent of hysterectomies performed in the two decades preceeding 1985. (There are no comprehensive statistics available for more recent times.)

Of these, prolapse, pregnancy, and PID constituted a significant number. In the latter two cases, hysterectomy is an extreme measure, but one that may be necessary to save a life.

Prolapse, however, is fortunately harmless most of the time. But this does not minimize the severe discomfort it can cause, nor does it compensate for the lifestyle changes it may impose. For example, a vaginal or uterine prolapse may interfere with sexual satisfaction, the ability to enjoy vigorous sports, or other aspects of an active life. It can cause bowel or bladder problems—even the formation of ulcers on the exposed portions of the cervix and uterus.

Here, a woman may decide to undergo a hysterectomy to ameliorate some of these symptoms. However, she may also opt for less radical solutions, such as pelvic floor exercises, estrogen creams, or pessaries first. In any case, this is a decision that can safely be left the patient depending on how she feels. It is *not* the place of the gynecologist to attempt to impose either a hysterectomy, or even a simple vaginal repair, on any woman whose symptoms are minimal or nonexistent.

Part 3

The Aftermath

I still hear stories every day from patients who say, "He wanted to clean me all out, so I wouldn't have to worry any more." "Clean me out" is a most disturbing expression. Does the doctor consider the uterus and ovaries dirty? Is the patient really cleaner without them?

I recently spent an hour at a teaching conference at Harvard Medical School. Problem patients were being presented for physicians' recommendations as to how they should best be treated. One patient was a 73-year-old man with prostate cancer. The urologist was extremely concerned with his therapy, as was the radiation therapist. The conversation went something like this:

Urologist: I think that a surgical approach might work, but I am really afraid that it would make him impotent.

Radiotherapist: Yes, but I'm not sure if the tumor can be well radiated because of its position. Radiation may not be a good choice for him.

Urologist: I am concerned. I wouldn't want him to lose his potency. Surgery in that area may ruin his sex life.

I almost had to pinch myself to make sure I wasn't dreaming. Here we have a patient with a spreading cancer who is 73 years old. His surgeon is carrying on and on about his sexuality. I'm not against sex, but where are the surgeons who defend women's sexuality when they are presented for castration (removal of the ovaries) in the hundreds of thousands? I have never heard so much as a peep from my surgical colleagues on their behalf . . .

No one ever seems to consider what the consequences might be for the woman and what it might do to her body image. I suppose if you are a man, it might seem that the loss of a uterus and ovaries is not important to a woman's sexuality. She can still have a sex life. And if her scar is well hidden, how could she ever know the difference? What they fail to realize is that women have feelings about their sexual organs, too. They may not be visible, but I still think that they are precious to us.

—Penny Wise Budoff, M.D.
No More Hot Flashes and Other Good News

8

Coping with the Aftermath

"It is important to understand that it is normal to mourn the loss of your reproductive capability. It is equally important to recognize that each woman will grieve in her own way."

—*Wanda Wigfall Williams*
Clinical Psychologist, 1982

"Instant" Menopause

Since the turn of the century, remarkable advances in medicine and technology have succeeded in *doubling* the life expectancy of American women who may now survive to an average age of approximately 80 years. This means that a woman can expect to spend a third of her life in the menopausal state. Thus there are presently 35 to 40 million postmenopausal women in the United States for whom attitudes and approaches to menopause have important reprecussions.

Is menopause a "disease" we need to "cure"? Dr. Wulf Utian argues in "The Fate of the Untreated Menopause": "As a result of my 20 years of research on menopause, I now believe that menopause may be considered an endocrinopathy"

If so, then what are the symptoms and, left untreated, what will be the adverse effects? What is the best "therapy"?

Undoubtedly, menopause *is* accompanied by several important physiologic changes (which not all women will experience equally). In addition, it cannot be debated that some of these changes are viewed as positive by the majority of women, that is, no more menstrual periods and no more fear of pregnancy. However, many of these changes are not positive, and they have varying degrees of serious impact on the older woman's health status.

For those women who undergo a natural menopause, physiologic changes occur very gradually and may be nearly unnoticeable, with a slight decline in ovarian function beginning in the late thirties or early forties and extending over a period of 15 or 20 years, until the actual cessation of menses. (See Figure 8.1.) However, no woman is as acutely aware of the changes in her body as the woman who has undergone an "instant menopause" brought on by a hysterectomy, especially when accompanied by an oophorectomy.

Furthermore, if the image of a woman in certain segments of our society is irreversibly tied to her reproductive capability, what does this say about her "worth" after menopause, and how do these attitudes impact on her psychological state? Certainly, from a historical perspective, menopause has been looked on in an unfavorable light. Here is a passage from an 1845 book entitled, *Treatise on the Diseases of Females:*

> Compelled to yield to the power of time, women now cease to exist for the species, and henceforward live only for themselves. Their features are stamped with the impress of age, and their genital organs are sealed with the signet of sterility.

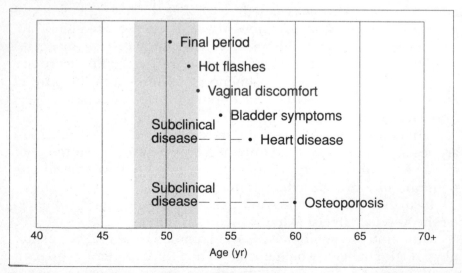

Figure 8.1 Graph of menstrual changes over time.

This chapter will attempt to place menopause in its proper perspective—to present an objective look at the mental and physical changes a woman may experience as a result of menopause, especially when accelerated by pelvic surgery. It will present some of the coping strategies a woman may employ to help her to continue to lead a healthy, long, and active life. Key to this discussion will be the role of hormone replacement therapy.

How Women Change with the "Change of Life"

Estrogens are vital organic compounds that are not the exclusive property of human women. Indeed, estrogens or receptors for estrogenlike compounds have been identified in men, lower animals, and even plants! That estrogens exert their influence throughout the human body (and not merely the genital tract) is proven by the presence of estrogen receptors in many organs, ranging from the skin to the brain and spinal cord, colon, pancreas, liver, adrenal glands, bladder, heart, and arteries. It is no wonder, then, that with menopause and the steady decline of ovarian estrogen production, the physiologic effects are seen and felt far and wide. (See Table 8.1.)

Ironically, the earliest effects, which are the ones that produce the most noticeable symptoms (e.g., hot flashes), are not necessarily the most lasting or the most serious long term. However, in the 1960s, it was for these symptoms that estrogen replacement therapy (ERT) was touted as the "fountain of youth" that would keep women "forever feminine." A decade later, ERT fell out of favor when several research studies, most notably those conducted by Drs. Ziel and Finkle and Dr. Mack, linked them to cancer. Today, hormone replacement therapy (in a modified form) is again being recommended. This time, however, it is not only advocated to ease the nonlife-threatening symptoms accompanying menopausal changes. It is now urged by many physicians that hormonal replacement therapy be considered by all postmenopausal women to stem the silent but deadly march of osteoporosis and cardiovascular disease. More will be said about this later in the chapter. For now, let's look at the early effects of estrogen depletion.

Table 8.1   Bodily changes with menopause

Organ	Symptom	Helped by Estrogen Repacement Therapy?
Uterus	Shrinkage in size and decreased muscle tone; weakening of support structures predisposing to prolapse.	Yes
Ovary	Cessation of ovulation and menstruation; loss of the ability to conceive.	No
Breasts	Reduction in size; weakening of support structures causing sagging of tissue.	Yes
Bladder	Thinning of tissues; increased susceptibility to infections and prolapse due to weakened support structures; causes increased frequency of urination and stress incontinence.	Yes
Nervous System	Hot flashes/flushes; depression; sleep disturbances; sexual dysfunction.	Yes
Skin	Increased thinning and dryness with associated itching.	Maybe
Hair	Increased dryness, thinning, and loss; possible facial hair development.	Maybe
Skeleton	Decreased bone mass with resulting osteoporosis.	Yes
Heart and Blood Vessels	Increased risk of cardiovascular disease, mainly attributed to changes in blood cholesterol.	Yes

Table 8.1   Bodily changes with menopause (continued)

Organ	Symptom	Helped by Estrogen Repacement Therapy?
Vulva	Shrinkage in size and fatty tissue; more susceptible to rashes and itching.	Yes
Vagina	Increased dryness and thinning of tissues; more susceptible to vaginitis and painful intercourse.	Yes

Hot Flashes and Flushes

These are the earliest and most commonly experienced effects of menopause. Experts estimate that as many as 75 to 85 percent of women undergoing menopause (naturally or via oophorectomy) will complain of hot flashes and flushes for at least a year, with up to 50 percent of women saying that they lasted for 5 to 10 years. Although not seeming to be a serious problem to those fortunate enough to be spared the effects, we know from the great numbers of women who seek medical attention for this problem that hot flashes and flushes may substantially interfere with the quality of a woman's life both during waking and sleeping hours. Most severely affected are women who experience "instant menopause," either via surgery or radiation.

A hot flash is the subjective premonition by the woman that she is about to experience a hot flush. Unlike flashes, hot flushes can be objectively measured. There is a definite change in temperature and pulse that is accompanied by the temporary, but sudden and profound, stretching of the blood vessels found in the skin of a woman's face, neck, and upper chest. This in turn causes increased blood flow to the area with profuse sweating. The underlying mechanism for these events seems to be a drop in estrogen levels that disrupts the hypothalamus—the body's "thermostat." For reasons as yet unknown, hot flushes seem to occur most commonly during the night, often disturbing a woman's rest. She may wake frequently, sometimes having to get out of bed to change her nightgown or the sheets. Some doctors have even hypothesized that the psychological symptoms some women complain of during menopause, such as fatigue, insomnia, irritability, difficulty concentrating, and depression may actually be a result of sleep deprivation secondary to hot flushes.

The American College of Obstetrics and Gynecology recently summarized the beneficial effects that numerous studies have concluded ERT has on hot flashes and flushes. They stated:

> Estrogen therapy effectively decreases the frequency and severity of subjective symptoms as well as the objective signs of menopausal flushes. With discontinuation of therapy, the symptoms may recur; gradually reducing the dose of estrogen in this situation, however, frequently minimizes the problem.

Progesterone, testosterone, and a blood pressure medication called *Clonidine* have also been demonstrated in some studies to alleviate hot flushes, although not as dramatically as estrogen. Estrogen remains the treatment of choice for this problem.

Vaginal Discomfort

As time passes, estrogen deficiency may also cause changes in the anatomy and physiology of a woman's vaginal area. The skin and hair covering the external structures (vulva) become thinner. Within the vagina, there are differences in the cells that comprise its structure and in the chemicals these cells produce. The vagina becomes drier, thinner, and shorter in some cases, thus making intercourse more uncomfortable for some women. In addition, it may be more easily injured and irritated. Because of chemical changes that occur, the premenopausal milieu that maintained a natural resistence to foreign bacterial invaders is now altered, thus causing a woman to be more susceptible to infections. The discharge and irritation that may result from trauma and infections related to menopause is called *atrophic vaginitis*. Some of the symptoms women notice with atrophic vaginitis include: burning, itching, white or clear discharge, and occasionally even bleeding.

If a woman remains sexually active during the menopausal years, these effects may be minimized or prevented. The mechanics of intercourse may keep the vagina from shortening. In addition, some doctors hypothesize that chemicals called *steroids* from the man's ejaculate may be absorbed by the woman thus resulting in an effect similar to estrogen replacement therapy.

As with hot flushes, estrogen replacement therapy has been found to be effective in reversing the vaginal changes associated with menopause. One study found that symptoms of vaginitis resolved in 89 percent of women, painful intercourse in 73 percent, and vaginal itching in 68 percent. Estrogen creams applied directly to the vagina are as effective as taking pills, and they may be more appealing to some women.

Bladder Symptoms

The cells of the bladder and the urethra (the structure leading from the bladder that allows the passage of urine from the body) are similiar to the vagina in their response to declining levels of estrogen. There may be irritation and increased susceptibility to infections due to thinning of these tissues. Some women also develop difficulties with incontinence when estrogen depletion causes them to lose muscle tone in their pelvic floor. As discussed in Chapter Seven, the pelvic floor may be stretched during childbirth and the bladder may prolapse into the vagina causing women to leak urine when they strain, cough, or laugh. Other estrogen-related changes have been observed having to do with the regulation of urine flow so that urine may remain in the bladder for prolonged periods again predisposing a woman to infections. ERT is effective in reversing many of the bladder symptoms of menopause and may help women to avoid hysterectomy from these causes.

The Skin

Several years ago, there was a commercial on televison advertising a dishwashing product in which a mother's and daughter's hands were displayed side by side. You weren't supposed to be able to tell the difference between these two women's ages until the camera panned to their faces. Thus far, science has been unable to prove dishwashing liquid has any beneficial effect on slowing the effects of aging on skin! Indeed, the skin contains estrogen receptors and is believed to be a major target of menopausal changes. However, it's also the most exposed organ of the body and subject to the greatest environmental influences. Therefore, it's difficult to determine whether the thinning, drying, and wrinkling of a woman's skin is actually from the cumulative effects of many years of daily wear and tear—all of those suntanning sessions, for example. It's likely that environmental exposures *along with* estrogen depletion contribute to the overall aging of a woman's skin. Unfortunately, estrogen replacement has not been established to be any more effective than dishwashing liquid in reversing these symptoms and is therefore not recommended. Here is what doctors at the Mayo Clinic have to say about ERT for skin changes:

> Estrogen is not a panacea for aging, and no available data prove that estrogen therapy confers cosmetic benefits.

The American College for Obstetricians and Gynecologists adds:

> The effects of estrogen replacement therapy on the skin . . . have not been clearly established. Until a beneficial cosmetic effect is demonstrated, the use of estrogen for this purpose cannot be recommended.

However, while I personally don't believe estrogen can restore *wrinkled* skin, I *do* believe that ERT begun early in menopause will prevent or retard skin *breakdown*.

Hot flushes, aging skin, and vaginal or bladder discomforts are the most frequent postmenopausal symptoms that bring women to the attention of their doctors. All of these are generally more flagrant when a woman has lost her uterus and/or ovaries during surgery. In the following sections, we take a look at conditions that develop more insidiously in postmenopausal women, with more profound implications.

Osteoporosis

Osteoporosis is a *major* health problem facing older women. At least 25 percent of all caucasian women will have had one or more fractures by the time they are 65. That's 1.5 million fractures per year! The cost of this condition, when you add up the dollars lost in income and those spent on medical care (hospitalization, surgery, physical therapy) and recovery in a nursing home is an incredible $6 to $10 billion annually. The costs in terms of personal damages cannot begin to be quantified when you consider that a woman in her late sixties or early seventies who fractures her hip may end up spending the rest of her life in an institution dependent on others for her needs and wants. Worse still, 2 out of every 10 victims of hip fracture die within a year because of complications.

Despite these sad and frightening statistics, we still haven't been able to seriously tackle this problem in postmenopausal women. Education regarding prevention is sorely lacking, and therapy once the disease has struck is also inadequate. Since 1940, we have known that estrogen replacement therapy is one of the few effective treatments for osteoporosis. Yet, for a variety of reasons, doctors and patients alike have neglected to aggressively pursue this. Today, only 10 percent of all postmenopausal women are on ERT for this condition.

Worse still is the contribution made by unnecessary hysterectomies to this public health crisis. In 1988, the results of a study made by Dr. Hreshchyshyn and his colleagues were published. They examined the effects of natural menopause as compared with hysterectomy and oophorectomy on spine and hip bones. The researchers confirmed that women who have undergone a hysterectomy had "significantly lower" bone densities than healthy women, even when their ovaries remained. One possible explanation for this is the observation that has been made that the ovaries of about one-third of women posthysterectomy cease to function one or two years after surgery. The decline in estrogen has been identified as a major contributing factor to osteoporosis. Furthermore, women who have their ovaries removed showed the most significant and the most rapid decline in bone densities of all groups, especially when their ovaries were removed at a younger age. Specifically, women who have their ovaries removed have *twice* the rate of bone loss as those who experience a natural menopause!

It's still an unsolved mystery as to why the lack of estrogen has such profound effects on a woman's skeleton because estrogen receptors have to this day never been definitely identified in bone. It may be estrogen's interaction with another hormone, called *parathyroid hormone*, and with calcium and vitamin D that initiates the loss in bone mass. While doctors remain unsure of the exact underlying mechanisms, what is clear is that osteoporosis is a *very serious* condition with the potential to cripple women. Therefore, a woman should realize the implications when she agrees to undergo a hysterectomy and/or oophorectomy and should *never* do so when other options exist.

A Bone Is a Living Thing

Because of its appearance, many of us tend to forget that bone is vital, dynamic living tissue. Like any other living tissue, it is constantly growing and changing. Bone consists of two types of cells that balance one another to accomplish this remodeling process. The first, called *osteoblasts*, are responsible for new bone development. The second, known as *osteoclasts*, mediate bone destruction. When we are babies, children, and teenagers, we experience a period of rapid bone growth which tapers off by the time we approach our mid-twenties. By our third decade, we experience a shift in bone development. Now, the balance tips toward a reduction in bone formation. Bone that is less dense is obviously more susceptible to injury from even day-to-day activities. When bone mass is decreased to the point that damage such as fractures may occur, *osteoporosis* is said to be present (see Figure 8.2).

Who Gets Osteoporosis?

Until menopause, rates of bone loss are similar in men and women. With estrogen decline, women undergo a rapid reduction in bone mass. Osteoporosis affects both the spongy types of bone found in the spine and wrists and the more compact bone found in the long bones of the hips. Relatively soon after estrogen depletion, osteoporosis afflicts the spongy bone, resulting in wrist fractures and spinal fractures. Interestingly, the latter may frequently cause no symptoms. The bones making up the spinal column, called *vertebrae*, may simply collapse without pain or injury. Eventually, a woman may notice a loss of height or a deformity in the upper back sometimes known as a *dowager's hump*. Later, as women reach their seventies, the compact hip bones become damaged to the point of fracture.

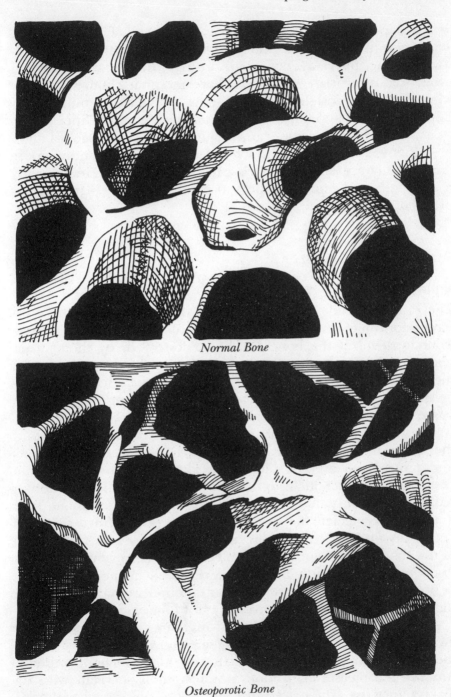

Normal Bone

Osteoporotic Bone

Figure 8.2   Normal bone versus osteoporotic bone—Bones with osteoporotic changes resemble swiss cheese.

Osteoporosis affects both men and women, but, since men start out with much denser bone to begin with, they are less likely to experience the ravages of osteoporosis. Most commonly affected are caucasian or Asian women who have never had children, women who are of short and slender build, those who have a family history of this condition and those with certain lifestyle habits. Specifically, women who have diets poor in calcium and high in alcohol and/ or caffeine; as well as women who smoke frequently and exercise infrequently are all at high risk for osteoporosis. Finally, early menopause, and especially surgical menopause, are prime causes of osteoporosis.

Making the Diagnosis

Bone Density Measurements

There are no easy, inexpensive, and therefore routine tests to screen for osteoporosis. Regular X rays will only reveal the disease when *one-third* of the bone has been destroyed. By then, other symptoms have already appeared. However, when women are at high risk of developing osteoporosis, they may be selected to undergo more accurate diagnostic tests for measuring bone density. Some of these include: *radiogrammetry, photodensitometry,* and *single-photon absorptiometry.* An explanation of these techniques is beyond the scope of this book. It will suffice to say that each has its limitations. Some are not suited for evaluating the portions of the skeleton most susceptible to osteoporotic damage. In addition, a measurement of bone density does not necessarily correlate with how strong bone actually is and thus how prone to fracture it may be. Finally, multiple tests may be necessary to present a true picture of the state of a woman's skeleton. For example, a woman may be losing bone mass rapidly, but still fall within the normal parameters of bone density for her age. However, another woman may have a slightly reduced bone mass, but may not be losing bone at all.

Other commonly used tests that measure spinal bone density include CAT scans and *dual-photon absorptiometry.* The problem with these tests is that, while they accurately measure bone mineral content, this measurement does not accurately correlate with actual fracture risk. The newest techniques use two X ray beams and

Major Risk Factors for Osteoporosis

You may already be in danger of developing osteoporosis if you . . .

- Are a woman
- Experienced menopause early
- Had a hysterectomy and/or oopherectomy
- Have never had children
- Smoke
- Drink alcohol
- Eat a diet high in caffeine and/or protein
- Eat a diet low in calcium and/or vitamin D
- Exercise rarely or not at all
- Exercise to the extreme of causing your menses to stop
- Are small in stature and slight in frame
- Suffer from thyroid or parathyroid disease
- Suffer from cancer
- Have diabetes mellitus
- Have anorexia nervosa
- Take certain medications, including: anticonvulsant medicines or steroids

measure both spine and hip bone densities. These, called, *quantified digital radiography* and *X ray absorptiometry* are quicker and more accurate.

In general, none of these tests is recommended routinely. However, while they have their flaws, they have proven to be useful in screening high risk patients and helping them to make a decision based on their bone density measurements as to whether they wish to start on ERT. Likewise, they are recommended for following the progress of patients who already have osteoporosis.

If diagnosis and treatment of osteoporosis are difficult, and the effects devastating, then clearly, *prevention* is the key. In the next section, we discuss ways in which women can reduce their risk of osteoporosis starting *long before* they attain menopause.

Prevention

Remembering these caveats can help women to start early in their battle against osteoporosis. First, bone depletion begins to exceed new bone creation when a woman is *only* in her thirties and not even beginning to think about menopause. Second, in the words of Dr. Bruce Ettinger, ". . . at this time there is no safe, effective means of restoring bone mass to normal once it has been depleted. . . ." Third, while a woman may have no control over some of her risk factors for osteoporosis, she can make lifestyle changes that will make a difference.

Changing Bad Habits . . .

"Coffin Nails"

One nurse I knew who worked in the emergency room at our hospital used to call cigarettes "coffin nails" because of the tremendous number of deaths he had seen attributable, at least in part, to smoking. "Every time they light one up they're just adding another nail to their coffin," he used to say. Scientists know that smokers past menopause are not only at greater risk for osteoporosis, but that their response to estrogen replacement is also poorer. This is not only true for bone mineral content. As we shall see in the next section, coronary artery disease is another major health concern for postmenopausal women. Smoking not only contributes to heart disease, but the beneficial effects ERT normally exerts on cholesterol levels are cut in half by smoking.

Dos and Don'ts of Diets

What you eat is as important as what you don't eat when it comes to osteoporosis. At a recent conference sponsored by the European Foundation for Osteoporosis and Bone Disease, experts made the following statement:

> Nutritional intake of elemental calcium is an absolute requirement for bone health, facilitating growth and consolidation and reducing bone loss after skeletal maturity has been reached. The threshold of calcium intake below which bone health is jeopardized varies at different stages of life. . . . It is likely that an adequate calcium intake is necessary for the maintenance of peak bone mass, but it is not known whether a high

calcium intake [in] adulthood can contribute to improvements in
bone mass. There is a need for studies to address the question of the
role of calcium supplementation in the third to fifth decades in women.

It is generally agreed that adequate calcium intake is essential to
healthy bones. The problem is, however, that most adult women
don't get enough calcium in their diets. This is true for a variety of
reasons. The major source of calcium is dairy. Unfortunately, some
women feel that dairy products are "too fattening." Others have an
intolerance to milk sugar, *lactose.* Ingesting milk or cheese causes
them to experience uncomfortable gastric problems, such as gas
and diarrhea. Others think you don't need to drink milk unless
you're a child. The end result is that half of all American women
over age 15 don't consume the minimum Recommended Daily
Allowance (RDA) for calcium of 800 milligrams. Worse still, as
women age, they don't absorb as much of the calcium that they
may take in. This is not only because an older woman's intestinal
tract is less efficient, but because vitamin D availability is also less.
   Vitamin D is intimately linked to calcium metabolism in the
human body. The chief source of this essential chemical is sunlight.
Humans synthesize vitamin D within their skin when exposed to
the sun, thus, when elderly women remain indoors for most of
their days, they may become deficient in this nutrient.
   Premenopausal women who are not pregnant should try to
consume 1,000 milligrams of calcium in their daily diets. The
sooner a woman increases her calcium intake the better because
bone growth is maximal before age 30. If a woman is past menopause, she needs to increase this to 1,500 milligrams per day.
(Whether diets high in calcium are really of major benefit to
women who already show the ravages of osteoporosis is controversial.
Certainly, it can't hurt, and it may help to heal fractures and/or
prevent further bone degeneration. As with anything else, be sure
not to overdo it, because excessive calcium may cause the formation of kidney stones.) In addition, 400 units of vitamin D are
needed every day. This can be accomplished either by being out in
the sun for at least 15 minutes at noontime or by drinking vitamin
D-fortified milk. Be careful about taking vitamin D supplements as
excess amounts can accumulate in body fat and become toxic.
   Appendix B provides a complete list of calcium-rich food
sources. You may be surprised to learn that many foods aside from
milk and cheese are high in this nutrient. These include: beans;

tofu; seafood; and green, leafy vegetables. Women also need to be aware of those substances that interfere with the availability of calcium to body tissues. Spinach, for one, contains a chemical called *oxalate* which binds calcium within the intestine. Diets high in fat and very high in fiber also decrease calcium absorption, as does excess amounts of zinc. Other substances cause calcium to be lost in the urine. Caffeine is one such culprit and is present in coffee, tea, cola drinks, and chocolate. Diets high in salt and protein have a similar effect. Try to cut down on alcohol consumption as well (two drinks per day or less). If all of this sounds like there's nothing safe left to eat, remember that the key to health is trying to have a balanced diet including moderate amounts of protein, carbohydrates, and vegetables with a special emphasis on dairy products.

Finally, don't forget that some medications disrupt calcium and/or vitamin D bioavailability. These include certain drugs taken to prevent seizures and tuberculosis as well as some antacids, blood pressure medications, and steroids used for asthma and arthritis. Women should check with their doctors concerning the specific medications they take and whether their dietary requirements may be affected.

"Couch Potato" Syndrome

When astronauts have been out in space where there is no gravity for their skeletons to work against, they have been shown to lose some bone mass. However, weight-bearing exercises are believed to stimulate formation of new bone. Thus it's a good idea to try to incorporate an exercise regimen into your lifestyle. Good gravity-resistive exercises include: walking, jogging, dancing, and light weight training. For example, almost every woman can safely walk for 30 minutes at least four times per week. Several words of caution: be very careful about the type of exercise you attempt if you already have osteoporosis. You don't want to place yourself at risk of falling and sustaining an injury or undertaking too vigorous a program for your present state of bone health. Consult your doctor first. Likewise, if you have been sedentary and are over age 35, be sure to have a check-up before beginning an exercise program. And, whatever age you are, begin gradually and build to a moderate pace.

Indeed, recent reports by research physiologist Barbara Drinkwater among others concerning female athletes raise some concerns for going to the other extreme when it comes to exercise. Bone density measurements for some young women who exercise intensely, such as ballet dancers or those women who are long distance runners, resemble those of 70-year-old women! This is believed to be because they stress themselves to the point of causing hormonal imbalances. Their menses stop and estrogen production declines just as if they are postmenopausal. Thus they begin to develop osteoporosis as if they are postmenopausal as well! Remember: slow and steady wins the race.

Estrogen Replacement Therapy for Osteoporosis

There is definite evidence that estrogen replacement therapy protects women against osteoporosis in several ways. First, if it is begun within five years of the start of menopause, ERT will *prevent* the loss of bone mass and subsequent fractures. For example, women begun on estrogen immediately after having an oophorectomy show almost complete cessation of bone deterioration.

Second, some doctors believe that even if some damage has already occurred, estrogen can arrest the process and even reverse some of the deterioration. According to Dr. Ettinger, "Estrogen reverses the bone resorption [thinning] rapidly, allowing the holes that have been formed in the bone to be filled in." It must be stressed, however, that not all doctors agree. Even if the remodeling of bone observed by Dr. Ettinger and others is proven out, these reverses are small. Once major changes in a woman's skeleton have taken shape, ERT cannot restore it to its normal form.

That is why prevention is centerstage with osteoporosis. Women begun on ERT soon after hysterectomy, oophorectomy or natural menopause will experience the most dramatic effects. It is unclear what benefits (if any) may be derived by women if they begin ERT more than five years after menopause. Many believe bone protection will commence at any stage and will continue for as long as a woman continues to take estrogen. Once she stops, however, the effects are unfortunately reversible. This makes ERT a long-term commitment (at least 10 years), the pros and cons of which must be evaluated by every woman and her physician individually. In

Chapter 9, we talk about how best to come to that decision for yourself.

Most of the studies that have been performed concerning ERT and osteoporosis have examined women taking a particular group of oral estrogen supplements called *conjugated equine estrogens*. It has been found that doses of 0.625 milligrams per day are safe and effective. Larger doses show no added benefit. And, it may even be possible to take smaller amounts under certain circumstances. One investigation by Dr. Genant and his associates found that the addition of 1,500 milligrams of calcium per day may cut the necessary dose of estrogen in half. Thus calcium and ERT may go hand-in-hand in protecting women from bone loss.

At present, we don't know enough about the impact other forms of estrogen therapy (i.e., creams and patches) may have on osteoporosis. Nor do we understand exactly *how* estrogen therapy accomplishes its effects. As we've said, no one has definitively proven that there are estrogen receptors in bone as there are in the skin, liver, and other organs affected by hormonal changes during menopause. We only know what we observe. That is, if estrogen replacement is begun, calcium absorption, vitamin D production, and calcitonin levels all become normal. (*Calcitonin* is a hormone that plays a role in bone turnover.) Clearly, much more research is needed in this area before the answers to many questions about the role of ERT in osteoporosis may be found.

Treatments on the Horizon

What if you can't or won't take estrogen and want to protect yourself from osteoporosis? Are there other forms of therapy for preexisting disease? What's new in the area of research and development for this condition? The following is a brief synopsis of alternatives to ERT.

Calcitonin

Like estrogen, calcitonin is a hormone which is believed to act against osteoporosis by retarding bone breakdown. Women taking calcitonin for 1 year show a 10 to 15 percent increase in bone density. Unfortunately, this effect may be short-lived, with no further improvements observed beyond this period, and regression when treatments are discontinued. In addition, calcitonin has several disadvantages which preclude its use for some women. It is extremely expensive, costing roughly $3,000 per year. It also must be administered by injection. (Researchers are in the process of creating a nasal spray.) Finally, because the most widely available form at present is derived from salmon, not humans, women may develop an immune response to calcitonin that renders it ineffective. On the positive side, synthetic calcitonin identical to the human substance has now been developed. This product promises to be more effective, especially in women intolerant to the salmon derivative. Currently, calcitonin is certainly a second choice after estrogen and should be reserved for those women who cannot be on ERT.

Fluoride

Believed by some scientists to be the sole treatment of osteoporosis in which new bone is actually *created*, fluoride use is controversial for a variety of reasons. First, the bone that is created may be more brittle than normal bone and thus may actually be *more prone to fractures!* Second, many women are unable to tolerate fluoride's unpleasant side effects, most notably gastric disturbances and inflamed joints. And, most significant, some of the latest reports seem to invalidate fluoride's efficacy entirely. Thus, this drug, (which is not FDA approved for osteoporosis), may soon become obsolete in favor of other, more promising therapies.

Thiazides (Diuretics)

These are a group of drugs also known as water pills that are most frequently used in the management of hypertension. It has been noted that women on thiazides seem to lose less calcium from their bodies, as is reflected by the calcium levels present in their urine. Whether this effect has any impact on preventing osteoporosis still remains to be seen, and investigations are currently underway.

Vitamin D

The role of vitamin D in the treatment of osteoporosis is very unclear. Some studies have shown its by-products (not the vitamin itself) to aid in calcium absorption and thus possibly to reduce bone loss and fractures. However, this evidence is far from conclusive. Furthermore, overdoses of vitamin D can be very harmful. In light of this, a cautious approach must be used with vitamin D. It's certainly a good idea to make sure your diet contains adequate amounts of both calcium and vitamin D, but not to consider it to be a definitive treatment for osteoporosis until we have more conclusive knowledge about its effects.

Parathyroid Hormone

There is a gland in every woman's body that is shaped like a butterfly with its wings wrapped around the windpipe in the neck. This gland is called the thyroid. The thyroid is important in the regulation of a woman's metabolism, somewhat like a thermostat regulates the rate at which a furnace burns fuel to keep energy levels optimal. Turn up the thermostat and the fire in the furnace flares, burning up more fuel and producing more energy. Likewise, an overactive thyroid speeds up the body's metabolism.

At each of the four corners of the "wings" or lobes of the thyroid, there are four tiny structures that make up the parathyroid gland. The parathyroid is instrumental in maintaining calcium balance in the body. Ninety-nine percent of the body's calcium is stored in our bones—the remainder circulates in the bloodstream and among our tissues that utilize it for such essential functions as conducting messages along our nerve pathways or contracting our muscles.

How much calcium is released from our bones versus how much is retained is governed by an intricate feedback system involving trace amounts of vitamin D and magnesium, but, mainly is the work of two opposing hormones. They are: calcitonin, which we have already alluded to, and parathyroid hormone (PTH). Calcitonin is produced in the thyroid while PTH comes from its namesake gland. PTH is responsible for removing calcium from the bone and adding it to the blood circulation while calcitonin has just the opposite effect. Thus it is not surprising that an overactive parathyroid gland would cause weakened bones more susceptible to fractures.

Scientists have observed that estrogen somehow keeps PTH levels in check, preventing depletion of calcium and loss of bone mass. Once women enter menopause, estrogen is no longer present to assure this effect. Furthermore, as we have already said, women tend not to take in as much calcium in their diets or absorb what is present as efficiently. The body senses this deficiency and compensates by increasing PTH levels and leaching calcium out of the bones. The end result, of course, is osteoporosis.

In studying PTH in the laboratory, a fascinating discovery was made. PTH in high doses does indeed cause bone breakdown. But, PTH in *low doses* increases bone formation, especially when combined with vitamin D! Limited studies, including those conducted by Dr. Reeve and his group, show substantial increases in the bone mass of women given this treatment regimen, but, it is not yet generally available and is still highly experimental. For now, this seems to offer a promising new avenue for the treatment of osteoporosis once we know more.

Etidronate

Etidronate, a chemical originally developed as a possible laundry detergent additive, is now showing promise as a new treatment for osteoporosis. According to a recent article in the *New England Journal of Medicine*, doctors nationwide conducted a two year investigation of the effects of etidronate on 429 women, all of whom had evidence of osteoporosis. Dr. Nelson Watts and his colleagues reported that those women placed on etidronate experienced an increase in spinal bone density and a decrease in new fractures as compared with women in the group not taking the drug. Indeed, the rate of new vertebral fractures was reduced by 50 percent in the women overall, and by as much as two-thirds in those women who had been most severely afflicted. Furthemore, this drug is comparable in cost to estrogen and calcitonin, has few side effects, and, being in pill form, is easy to take. Overall, the authors of this study call etidronate "a welcome addition to the therapeutic options for osteoporosis."

Finally, researchers are investigating a means of combining a variety of substances and medications including estrogens, calcitonin, PTH, and/or vitamin D to attempt to restore the physiologic balance between bone formation and decomposition. This is called *coherence therapy.*

For now, the best way to overcome osteoporosis is to avoid it entirely. What that means is to stress the building of strong bones from a young age through diet, exercise, *and the avoidance of unnecessary hysterectomy or oophorectomy.* If a woman is at high risk of succumbing to osteoporosis or has already begun to show telltale signs, she should seriously consider estrogen therapy. To date, it is the only proven intervention that stops, and may even reverse, the serious declines in bone mass brought on by aging.

Another reason women should seriously consider ERT has to do with the effects menopause seems to have on the cardiovascular system. In the next section, we take a look at coronary artery disease.

Heart Disease

Arteriosclerotic disease, which causes a narrowing of the blood vessels supplying necessary oxygen to the heart, brain, and other major organ systems of the body, is responsible for the deaths of *one out of every two* Americans. That makes it the most significant health problem facing us today, including all forms of cancer. Interestingly, it has been discovered that women seem to be protected from the ravages of arteriosclerotic disease until they enter menopause, after which their rate of death and disease catches up to men's. As you might imagine, this has significant implications for the woman considering having a hysterectomy and/or oophorectomy.

Arteriosclerosis: Takes a Lickin'. . . Can It Keep on Tickin'?

The heart is an incredible feat of engineering. A muscular structure containing four chambers, it contracts an average of 60 to 80 times per minute every minute of our lives from the time we are still within our mother's uterus to the second we die. With each contraction, blood is forced from the top two chambers into the bottom two chambers and out into the blood vessels which will carry it to all parts of our body. Within this blood are chemicals vital to the maintenance of life, including oxygen, which is the basic fuel for our daily activities. Like any other organ, the heart itself requires oxygen and the *coronary arteries* are the blood vessels responsible for servicing the heart's needs.

Arteriosclerosis begins when a type of fat called *cholesterol* is present in the circulation in excessive amounts. Cholesterol accumulation (among other factors) can cause damage to the vessel walls. These damaged areas attract a particular type of blood cell called *platelets* which stick to the area and begin to stimulate the

Not All Cholesterol Is "Created Equal"

What is cholesterol?

Cholesterol is a waxy substance that humans both manufacture and ingest. It is a vitally important building block for the body, playing a role in the manufacture of hormones, vitamins, and digestive chemicals, to name a few.

Where does cholesterol come from?

It is found all over the body, although it is synthesized and stored in the liver. (Dietary sources of cholesterol are found only in animal products, not in plants.) When cholesterol is present to excess, it can clog blood vessels, causing cardiovasular disease.

What's the difference between "LDL" and "HDL" cholesterol?

Not all cholesterol is created equal. "LDL" stands for "low density lipoprotein" and "HDL" signifies "high density lipoprotein." A lipoprotein is a kind of envelope with a protein coat that carries fat and cholesterol through the bloodstream. LDLs contain large amounts of cholesterol that are then deposited in the arterial walls, whereas HDLs contain only small amounts of cholesterol, which they transport away from body tissues to be excreted. Therefore, high levels of LDL cholesterol are associated with an increased risk of coronary artery disease. A high HDL cholesterol is considered to be "heart healthy."

What's a normal cholesterol level?

Desirable cholesterol counts for most laboratories are:

> TOTAL CHOLESTEROL: BELOW 200 mg/dl
> LDL CHOLESTEROL: BELOW 130 mg/dl

buildup of muscle cells in the lining of the artery. Eventually, the blood vessel wall becomes narrower and narrower, thus restricting the passage of oxygen-rich blood. When this happens to the vessels supplying the heart, it's called coronary artery disease.

When this process develops gradually, the heart learns to compensate for ordinary activities. However, under conditions of physical or emotional stress, the heart may require additional energy (and therefore oxygen) which it cannot receive due to the physical limitations of the narrowed arteries. Lack of oxygen causes chest pain, which is known as *angina pectoris*. This is why, classically, people experience angina when they are upset or exerting themselves in some manner. If a total blockage of a major artery ensues, the portion of heart muscle supplied by that vessel will die. This is what happens during a heart attack.

Likewise, when this process of decreased supply of oxygen to meet the demand occurs in the blood vessels of the brain, *transient ischemic attacks* (TIAs) or "mini-strokes" take place. Complete blockage or rupture of a blood vessel within the brain is the cause of a stroke. Together, the effects of narrowed blood vessels throughout the heart, brain, and circulation are categorized under the title cardiovascular disease.

Damage to the heart may be detected by a number of diagnostic tests, including the electrocardiogram which measures the electrical activity of the heart and can be performed at rest or when the body is subjected to a controlled but stressful situation. The value of stress tests in women before menopause is very controversial because results have been very inconsistent. CAT scans, MRIs, and other methods may be used to diagnose suspected strokes.

Who Is at Risk?

Women in general seem to have a 10- to 12-year reprieve from the onset of cardiovascular disease, but they catch up rapidly once they enter their middle years. Perhaps the largest and most famous investigation of cardiac disease, the Framingham Heart Study, was undertaken over 40 years ago and is still going on today. According to the data collected in Framingham, Massachusetts,

> . . . after 44 years of age, arteriosclerotic disease rises in women at the same rate as in men, and women have the same number of new cardiovascular disease events.

Women, like men, place themselves at greater risk for heart attack and stroke if they smoke, or allow themselves to become overweight by eating a high fat diet and leading a sedentary lifestyle. The two main medical conditions that also predispose to cardiovascular disease are high blood pressure and diabetes.

Promoting Wellness

As with osteoporosis, prevention is possible. In Appendix B, you will find information on heart-healthy diets. The major emphasis is a reduction in your salt, cholesterol, and fat intake. Salt makes the body retain fluid and this fluid expands the blood volume. More blood pumping through the same space within an artery (or a narrowed artery when there is arteriosclerosis) causes the blood pressure to rise. This is easy to envision if you think of water contained within a hose. When you either turn up the water or narrow the hose, the pressure increases.

The American Heart Association, nutritionists, and others have advocated that Americans reduce the amount of fat and cholesterol in their diets. Remember that the two are not the same. Cholesterol is strictly an animal product. However, while vegetables are always free of cholesterol and nearly always low in fat, this is not always the case. Certain vegetables, like avocados and coconuts are completely free of cholesterol but extremely high in harmful fats. Likewise, fish is generally preferred over red meat in terms of a lower cholesterol content and the presence of certain so-called cardioprotective omega-3 fatty acids. However, shellfish is nearly as damaging as red meat. Thus it is important to familiarize yourself with food labels and types. Armed with this knowledge, you can balance your diet with foods that are low in cholesterol or fats and high in substances, such as fiber, which may actually reduce cholesterol levels. (Again, the information in Appendix B will help you to achieve this goal.)

Exercise is also vitally important. It strengthens the heart both directly and indirectly (for instance, by lowering blood pressure). When a woman runs 10 to 15 miles per week or walks twice as much, she will experience a significant increase in her HDL cholesterol levels after about three to four months. Furthermore, aerobic exercises in particular seem to add 10 years to a woman's life. Cardiopulmonary fitness tests conducted on sedentary women versus active women showed astonishing results. A 40- to 49-year-old woman who worked out regularly was in better shape than inactive women aged 30 to 39. Weight lifting is important in preparing a woman's body for aerobic activities but in and of itself does not show similar effects in terms of improving cardiac fitness.

Walking, cycling, and swimming are activities nearly all women can enjoy and profit from.

Menopause and Heart Disease

Why should menstruating women have any advantage when it comes to heart disease? Scientists are still unsure, although the obvious clue is that estrogen levels decline dramatically once a woman stops menstruating. When estrogen supplements are given to women past menopause, changes occur in their cholesterol levels. Specifically, levels of so-called good cholesterol (protective against coronary disease), known as high-density lipoprotein cholesterol (HDL), rise while harmful low-density lipoprotein cholesterol (LDL) levels fall. Another potential factor may concern the content of a woman's blood pre- and postmenopause. Many women are mildly anemic during their menstruating years. The relatively thinner concentration of their blood as compared with a man's or a menopausal woman's may make it less prone to stagnating and thus forming a blood clot. In addition, thinner blood provides less resistance to arterial walls and results in lower blood pressure. Lower blood pressure places less stress on the heart and reduces the risk of cardiovascular disease.

Finally, there may be one hypothetical cause of heart disease unique to hysterectomy-induced menopause. The uterus produces a substance called *prostacyclin* which is critical to blood circulation. Specifically, prostacyclin inhibits clotting while dilating or widening blood vessels. Once the uterus is no longer present, prostacyclin levels drop. Coronary artery disease may develop more easily in the presence of more viscous blood within a narrower vessel.

Whatever the specific mechanisms involved, postmenopausal women are at definite risk of succumbing to heart attacks and strokes. Furthermore, women who undergo so-called surgical menopause through the removal of their uterus and ovaries have a risk of arteriosclerosis that develops earlier *and* to a more serious degree than women undergoing natural menopause. Most, but not all, of the evidence now shows that estrogen replacement therapy may restore a woman to her premenopausal state with regard to heart disease risk.

The Heart and Estrogen Replacement Therapy

If you are at all familiar with birth control pills, you may be wondering how the estrogen in ERT can protect a woman against cardiovascular disease when the risk of this very same condition is the major harmful consequence of estrogen-containing oral contraceptives. It seems that the answer to this puzzle lies with the fact that ERT relies on totally different types of estrogens (natural versus synthetic) in completely different dosages. According to the American College of Obstetricians and Gynecologists, ". . . estrogen replacement therapy has not been associated with an increased incidence of stroke, embolism, or thrombophlebitis. . . ." Still not convinced? Let's take a look at the evidence concerning postmenopausal women, estrogen, and heart disease.

First, it's important to examine how estrogen replacement might impact on the risk factors for heart disease we have already highlighted, especially cholesterol levels, smoking, obesity, and high blood pressure. Unfortunately, with the exception of its effects on lipids (cholesterol), there is a paucity of data available.

In 1952, Dr. Barr provided the first evidence that women taking oral estrogens had a change in the makeup of their cholesterol. There seemed to be an increase in the HDL component with a decrease in LDL, thus improving these women's risk of developing cardiovascular problems. While it has remained controversial whether *total* cholesterol levels remain the same or decrease, numerous subsequent studies have borne out Dr. Barr's original finding that oral estrogen tips the HDL/LDL balance in favor of the heart. As Dr. Ettinger points out,

> . . . larger doses may reduce the total cholesterol and increase the high-density lipoprotein [HDL] by as much as 10%. Although these changes seem relatively minor, reducing a cholesterol level of 250mg/dl [normal levels are considered to be values under 200 for most labs] by 25 mg/dl should result in a 50% reduction in arteriosclerotic risk.

It is important to note, however, that it is not as clear how other forms of estrogen may influence lipids, particularly those estrogens that are not processed through the liver (which manufactures, stores, and removes cholesterol). Furthermore, when progesterone is added to the estrogen replacement regimen, some of the heart-protective effects may be negated. This seems to depend on what type of progesterone is prescribed by your physician, so be sure to ask about this when considering ERT.

Finally, smoking also alters the effects of estrogens on cholesterol levels. While both smokers and nonsmokers appear to reap the benefits of taking estrogens, smokers can expect to experience only half the response in their lipid levels as nonsmokers.

What about ERT if you are overweight or have high blood pressure? These are again contraindications to estrogen-containing oral contraceptives. Does the same apply here? Apparently, the answer is "no." The limited work that has been done does appear to show that women who are overweight and who are begun on ERT actually *lose* weight, while normal-sized women do not gain weight. Even more interesting is the fact that women past menopause who do *not* begin ERT actually *gain* weight.

There does not seem to be an association between either high blood pressure or formation of blood clots and ERT. However, convincing evidence links birth control pills with all of the above. Therefore, your doctor may be reluctant to prescribe ERT if you are overweight, have had a blood clot, or hypertension problem. These factors must be considered on an individual basis while doctors continue to seek conclusive answers through additional research.

Thousands of women on estrogen have now been studied in an attempt to determine whether they actually do have fewer heart attacks, strokes, and/or deaths associated with heart disease. Nearly a score of reports have been published, with almost half finding a clear reduction in the risk of cardiac disease for women using estrogens and another fourth finding neither an advantage nor a disadvantage. These studies looked at women from all walks of life, including nurses, residents of a retirement community, and participants in a health maintenance organization, to name a few. All in all, most doctors conclude from weighing all the evidence that taking estrogen may even have dramatically beneficial effects, lowering the number of fatal and nonfatal heart attacks by 50 percent! If a woman has had her ovaries removed, the arguments are even stronger. By some estimates, the death rate is *six to seven times higher* when estrogen supplements are not taken. (Figure 8.3 compares the heart disease–related death rates in users versus

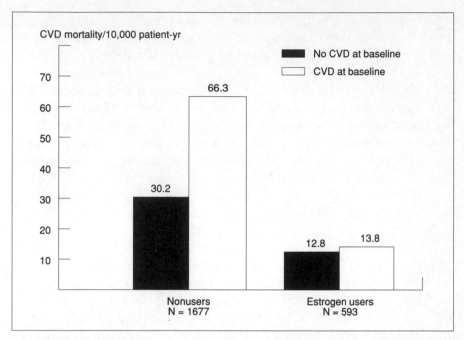

Figure 8.3   Comparison of heart disease–related deaths in users versus nonusers of estrogen replacement.

nonusers of ERT, according to research from the American Heart Association.)

Thus far, we've looked only at the purely physical effects women may anticipate once they undergo menopause. We've seen how these effects can unfortunately be accelerated and exacerbated by premature menopause brought on by removal of the ovaries and (sometimes) the uterus. But what about the less easily identified and quantified psychological effects some women have reported? From my experience, there seems to be a genuine and serious emotional aftermath as well.

The Emotional Fallout

Hysterectomy, oophorectomy, and its inevitable consequence, menopause, have all been cited as the cause of such psychological symptoms as: depression, anxiety, mood swings, decreased memory, impaired concentration, insomnia, fatigue, and decreased sexual desire. Some of these, as we alluded to earlier, may be as a direct result of physiologic (hormonal) changes—most notably hot flushes.

It has been observed that so-called REM (rapid eye movement) sleep, the most restful type of sleep, is decreased and disrupted by the occurrence of nocturnal hot flushes. It comes as no surprise, then, that women who awaken several times a night in a profuse sweat suffer from insomnia, fatigue, and the various consequences of sleep deprivation, such as difficulty concentrating or remembering as well as general moodiness. Estrogen, you will recall, as well as progesterone, will help if the underlying problem is purely physical and *not* as a result of a more deep-seated regret or ambivalence toward the loss of one's uterus.

Two common and more extensively studied psychological symptoms linked to hysterectomy and menopause are depression and sexual dysfunction. The chance of developing these conditions is a serious concern raised by women both before and after they undergo hysterectomy. Thus it is important that we carefully examine both with respect to how commonly they actually strike, and in terms of what can be done to minimize any damaging effects they may cause.

Depression

In 1941, the first reports of depression following pelvic surgery were published in the scientific literature by Dr. Lindemann. Later, a term was even coined for it: *post-hysterectomy syndrome.* Various studies pointed to a higher rate of admissions to psychiatric hospitals for women who had undergone a hysterectomy as well as a generally higher rate of emotional problems (two to three times higher) among women experiencing the removal of their uterus as compared with women having their gallbladders removed. Mental illness, it seemed, was a common side effect of hysterectomy, afflicting by some estimates as many as 70 percent of women postoperatively! Yet, this knowledge did not deter physicians from subsequently performing millions of these operations each year.

More recently, these conclusions have been challenged in some circles, and the subject has become more controversial. However, many hysterectomy patients that I have seen tell me the story of severe loss—of grief over the loss of an organ of their body. Because of this, I routinely counsel patients contemplating this surgery and ask them how they would feel if they had a hysterectomy. Instead of having patients tell me that they really don't know how they might feel, I get one of two answers. Some patients say that they will experience significant grief and that they don't want to lose their uterus—even if it is causing them pain, even if it is malfunctioning; even if there is the possibility that less invasive surgery now (i.e., myomectomy) might mean more surgery later. Certainly these patients will experience a significant loss if faced with a hysterectomy. However, some women with whom I discuss the possibility of uterine conservation reply that they don't feel that it's necessary to save their uterus. After all, they argue, what do they need it for? They're not going to have children. They're experiencing a troublesome problem, such as a large fibroid, that may continue to cause problems at a later date, and they want to have the uterus removed. These women are probably not going to become depressed because they want to have the surgery. Thus it's my judgment that the causation of this depression is a mind-set. And, from my experience, 8 out of 10 women *want their uterus preserved!*

Therefore, it's vitally important for an individual woman contemplating hysterectomy to consider that she may become depressed and to be aware of what factors increase her risk.

The next section deals with these issues and discusses what coping strategies she may have at her disposal to assist her.

How Will I Feel?

Joan is a 42-year-old mother of two grown sons. When Joan's second son was born, she was treated briefly for a bout of postpartum depression. Married to a truck driver who is often on the road for long periods of time, Joan finds herself with frequent slots of empty time on her hands now that her job of full-time wife and mother is not as demanding. Despite the necessity of sacrifices and strict budgets, Joan says she and her husband both felt it was more important for her to be home for the children and to manage the household than to have a career of her own. Except for recent times, Joan always felt that she was "too busy" to get involved with outside activities, such as charitable works or the PTA.

Two months ago, Joan underwent a hysterectomy with removal of both of her ovaries for a fibroid tumor. Her gynecologist had told her that he was alarmed by its unusually large size and advised that surgery be scheduled immediately. Joan and her husband heard the words "large tumor" and agreed that she would have the surgery scheduled two weeks later.

Because of the nature of his job, Joan's husband is not really available to help her with some of the work around the house she still feels incapable of resuming. Furthermore, she is concerned that he is distancing himself from her, for example, by deliberately volunteering for overtime and for particularly extensive road trips.

Lately, especially when no one is home, Joan finds herself lying in bed until noon and hanging around the house in her nightgown. She feels listless and seems to "cry at the drop of a hat." She feels very unattractive and finds that she is sometimes grateful that her husband has found other things besides her to occupy himself with.

Some women do become clinically depressed after a hysterectomy. Therefore, *all* women should think twice about the need for their hysterectomy. They should weigh any available alternatives, and take into consideration how they will feel when it's all over. If a woman has made a well thought out, well-informed decision and has allowed herself and her family adequate time and resources to prepare for hysterectomy; if she feels that having the operation is the best choice in her situation, she will significantly minimize any depression.

Joan's story highlights some of the risk factors and symptoms associated with post-hysterectomy syndrome. First, she had a history of a previous bout with depression after the birth of her son. She has opted for a very traditional role—one in which childrearing was central to her concept of herself. Now, Joan's children are grown and she must readjust and consider how she will spend the rest of her life. Right now, she is bored, with too much time on her hands. Furthermore, Joan's partner is both physically and emotionally distant from her. He seems to view her along traditional lines as well, and both Joan and her husband may have certain notions about hysterectomy and sexuality that are influencing their attitudes and behavior. Finally, Joan had the operation within a month of her initial doctor's visit, which left them little time to be properly educated or emotionally prepared. All of these factors have resulted in Joan clearly demonstrating some of the symptoms of depression, including: feelings of listlessness, sadness, decreased sexual desire, and a disinterest in day-to-day life.

Depression: A Self-Help Guide

The following is a list of the major symptoms indicating depression, according to the American Psychiatric Association. If you answer "yes" to at least five of the questions and have had these feelings for at least two weeks, you should consider seeking help for your depression.

1. *Are you in a depressed or irritable mood* most of the day, nearly every day, as indicated by your own feelings or as observed by others?

2. *Do you have a markedly diminished interest or pleasure in all, or almost all, activities* most of the day, nearly every day, as indicated by your own feelings or the observation by others that you are apathetic? Have you noticed that you don't feel much better, even temporarily, when something good happens?

3. *Have you experienced a significant weight loss or weight gain* (e.g., more than 5 percent of your body weight in a month), or a *decrease or increase in appetite nearly every day?*

4. *Do you suffer from insomnia or excessive sleepiness* nearly every day? Are you waking up two hours (or more) earlier in the morning than usual?

5. *Have others noticed that you are excessively agitated or lethargic* nearly every day?

6. *Do you feel fatigued—without any energy—*nearly every day?

7. *Do you have feelings of worthlessness or excessive or inappropriate guilt* nearly every day?

8. *Do you feel unable to concentrate, or indecisive,* nearly every day, in your own judgment or by the observation of others?

9. *Do you have recurrent thoughts of death* (not just fear of dying), *recurrent suicidal ideas* (without a specific plan)? *Have you made a suicide attempt or a specific plan for commiting suicide?*

Depression is a common side effect of hysterectomy. Fortunately, talking with a therapist and/or medications are extremely helpful in curing the depression. If you or your loved one is experiencing these symptoms, *seek help*.

Reprinted with permission from the American Psychiatric Association: *Diagnostic and Statistical Manual of Mental Disorders, Third Edition, Revised,* Washington, D.C. American Phsychiatric Association, 1987.

David Youngs and Thomas Wise, two experts in the field of psychological aftereffects following elective hysterectomy, tell us that the main issues for women facing hysterectomy include: the loss of reproductive function, the loss of menstrual function, and threats to sexual function. Women who consider hysterectomy before they have completed their families are bound to be severely depressed once this is no longer a possibility for them. And, even women for whom menstruation may have been fraught with problems, may express depression once they no longer experience what most women view as a natural, valuable, and uniquely female function. But, of all the risk factors that have been cited to cause postoperative depression, one of the most common revolves around a woman's fear of sexual changes. In research that studied women's anxiety related to hysterectomy, the women who became depressed afterward were those who believed that hysterectomy would make them fat, prematurely old, less interested in sex, and less desirable to their husbands. Thus how a husband deals with his wife's surgery is just as important to her mental health and self-esteem as are her own feelings. In an article published in the journal, *Psychosomatics,* Drs. Lalinec-Michaud and Engelsmann write:

> A woman who is insecure about her attractiveness is more prone to expect that her husband might lose interest in her following the removal of her womb. Indeed, the husband's reaction has a strong influence on the woman during this sensitive period of time . . . strong support from the spouse may greatly facilitate a healthy rehabilitation period.

Unfortunately, men have been known to reject their wives and marriages have broken up more often as a result of this surgery than, for example, gallbladder operations. Clearly, both men and women have to understand what's happening and come to grips with their feelings to avoid these consequences.

What You Can Do If You Need a Hysterectomy
Experts believe that you can avoid or minimize posthysterectomy depression if you heed the following guidelines.

Be sure to tell the gynecologist what you want. Make sure you trust your gynecologist and get a second opinion whenever possible so that you are comfortable that having a hysterectomy is the course you wish to pursue in the treatment of your gynecologic problem. If you truly don't want to lose your uterus under any circumstances, seek that second opinion with a physician who is sensitive and attuned to alternate methods (methods which help women to avoid hysterectomy whenever it is at all feasible). Research has shown that women suffering from nonlife-threatening problems (which might have been solved another way?) were much more likely to become depressed than those who expressed a profound sense of relief that a dreaded condition (e.g., cancer) was now behind them. Certainly, hysterectomy will solve the *medical* problems and the *anatomical* defects in a woman with fibroids, for instance, *but the body is more than a uterus!* The body is more fundamentally a human being with a human mind and emotions. Therefore, the gynecologist has to be concerned with finding out from a woman exactly what this surgery would mean to her, and to understand that even if a woman is prepared to take certain (nonlife-threatening) risks to preserve her self-image, he must respect and comply with her feelings. As long as a woman *understands* that the alternative to hysterectomy she has selected may not offer a permanent solution or a 100 percent cure, then *she is entitled to make the choice.*

To sum up, here are the words of Youngs and Wise:

> Social, psychological, and even cultural aspects of gynecologic surgery inevitably involve three principal individuals—the patient, her family, and the physician. Each plays a critical role in the successful outcome of any surgical treatment. A healthy comfortable relationship among all participants provides the best insurance against misunderstanding, regret, and subsequent untoward psychological sequelae.

Researchers Hackett and Weisman further reinforce my admonition concerning the absolute necessity of finding an understanding physician:

> . . . unless it is understood that the interpersonal dimension operates within both patient and doctor, the patient is apt to be considered identical with the diseased organ and the surgeon a totally disengaged technician.

Get "the facts, ma'm, just the facts." It's important that you and your partner sit down with your doctor or nurse and receive a clear explanation of the operation, the recovery period, and any long-term side effects. Review any concerns you may have and dispel any erroneous fears based on what you may have heard from others. Be sure that you ventilate all of your feelings and get *concrete and realistic* answers to all your questions. Various studies have shown that even women who did receive information before their operations may not have benefited very much. In follow-up interviews, they complained that the advice was too broad. For example, they may have been told not to lift anything heavy, but not exactly what the weight limitations were or for how long they should maintain the restriction. Or, women were sung the praises of hysterectomy ("you'll be a new woman in six weeks") when their recovery actually took much longer in many cases. In addition, discussions were sometimes described as too short, with too much information presented for them to assimilate in one sitting. Try to have several conversations with your doctor or nurse and make sure you keep in contact until all of your questions have been answered. Finally, even health professionals may be reluctant to bring up the topic of sex, so don't you be. Remember, uncertainty in this area was one of the most frequently cited risk factors for depression.

Allow yourself time to do "the work of worrying." Unless it's an emergency, take time to prepare yourself for the surgery—emotionally and physically. You may not think that having a hysterectomy will represent a big change in your life but it very well may, and people generally need time to "psyche themselves up," as has been proven by studies comparing rates of depression for women who knew at least a month ahead that they were going to lose their uterus as compared to women who did not. Consider the advice of Dr. Lalinec-Michaud and Dr. Engelsmann:

> Women having a hysterectomy after short notice experienced a significantly greater pre- and postoperative depressive morbidity. It is conceivable that women need some "mourning time" to adjust to the thought of an important intervention such as hysterectomy, which is perceived as a loss and a threat to the integrity of self-concept. Allowing sufficient time prior to the operation, when possible, would help facilitate better pre- and post-operative adjustments.

Have frank and open discussions with your partner concerning what this surgery represents to both of you. Don't minimize or deny your feelings. If you fear that you may somehow become less attractive or less sensuous, gaining reassurance from your partner that he doesn't feel this way can make all the difference. If your partner worries that you may be "altered"; that because you can no longer get pregnant you're no longer as appealing somehow, or that you'll lose interest in sex, it's imperative that you work this out. You may both need to seek professional help either to set the facts straight or to cope with these feelings.

Realize that you are not alone and that help is available in the form of support groups (see Appendix A), psychotherapy, and medication, should you become depressed. Remember that feeling depressed from time to time is quite normal. It only turns into actual pathology when these feelings are so severe and prolonged that they interfere with your ability to deal with daily life. If you find that you are feeling sad, worthless, anxious, unattractive, ill, helpless, or hopeless (especially to the point of contemplating suicide) and if these feelings pervade every facet of your life from work to leisure for two weeks or more, it's time to seek help.

Keep active and lead a healthy lifestyle. This is generally good advice for any situation. Specifically here, however, if a woman has other diversions and interests not tied to mothering, she may not feel all is lost when her uterus is lost. In addition, from a practical point of view, exercising regularly will help you to avoid the weight gain you may fear to be a consequence of hysterectomy. Furthermore, exercise increases the levels of chemicals in the brain called *beta endorphins.* These are known to reduce pain and increase one's feelings of general well-being. Plenty of rest and good nutrition is also essential to dealing with any stress and hysterectomy is no exception. High-protein foods, such as milk, also improve one's sleep and sense of well-being. In addition, avoiding the urge to take solace in empty calories avoids making depression worse through weight gain.

Sexuality: How Much Psychology? How Much Physiology?

Roughly 40 percent of women report a decrease in sexual response after hysterectomy. Contributing to these troublesome statistics are a variety of physical and emotional factors. As we've pointed out in the previous section, issues concerning sexuality are often the prime suspects in posthysterectomy depression. Women (or their partners) who *believe* they will experience sexual problems actually *have* more sexual problems as the result of a self-fulfilling prophecy. It's vitally important that women and their sexual partners confront their fears and raise their concerns in this area in order to minimize this effect. Ellen and her husband had tremendous difficulties in this area after her hysterectomy:

When I was 38 I had a hysterectomy for severe bleeding. I was being so tortured by my periods, that I didn't even think about any "down side" to the surgery. Something else was going on in the back of my husband, Ed's, mind, however. Naturally, I didn't think much about Ed's lack of sexual advances immediately after my operation. After all, he was just being cautious and considerate. The doctor had told us to avoid intimacy during the recovery period until I returned for my postoperative examination.

It was after I was given the "green light" that I noticed something was wrong. The first time, it really hurt. I told myself that I must have been nervous. Still, I could see that there was a change in Ed's manner and behavior. He must also be nervous, I mused.

I decided to discuss the matter with my gynecologist, since I was concerned that something might have gone wrong with the surgery. He told me that absolutely nothing had gone wrong with the surgery and that having your uterus removed had nothing at all to do with sex. Sex, he said, was in your mind not in your uterus. He told me not to listen to what other women said about how their sex lives changed after hysterectomy. These were "old wive's tales" and I was a "modern woman." He said that I was probably sending subliminal messages to my husband which were affecting his performance as well.

In other words, it was "all in my head"; it was all "my fault"; it was from a mythology built up by women and the sooner I realized all of this, the sooner I'd "get well." In fact, what I discovered was that it was my husband's fears and beliefs that were at the root of the problem. He came from a very old-fashioned family and his value system prevented him from enjoying sex with a "neutered woman." Unfortunately, he did not consciously confront his feelings beforehand, and it took us some time to work through this in therapy afterward.

Ellen's gynecologists' words sound very reminiscent of those of W. Gifford-Jones, M.D., author of the book, *What Every Woman Should Know about Hysterectomy.* In it he says:

> Gynecologists would have stopped doing this operation years ago except where it was life-saving if a significant number of their patients ended up in the psychiatrist's hands. The same thing applies to cases one hears about where women have a change of heart sexually toward their partners. Lamentably, many problems exist in the bedrooms of the nation long before a hysterectomy is required. *To some women, the operation therefore presents an excellent out. Yet it is impossible to change a healthy woman's posture towards sex, and women who have always enjoyed sex will have the same liking for it after the operation.* [Emphasis added.]

It's easy to "blame" a woman for what may be a natural decline in sexual interest and activity with the approach of middle age, especially if she's undergone menopause or hysterectomy. In actual fact, the renowned Dr. Kinsey discovered in his research on human sexual response that *both men and women experience parallel decreases in sexual interest* beginning around the fourth or fifth decades of life, and these were unrelated to a woman's hormones. A century before, Dr. Colombat L'Isere had pronounced sex dead after menopause:

> It is the dictate of prudence to avoid all such circumstances as might tend to awaken any erotic thoughts in the mind and reanimate a sentiment that ought rather to become extinct . . . in fine, everything calculated to cause regret for charms that are lost, and enjoyments that are ended forever.

Today, by contrast, many postmenopausal women who now see themselves as free of the concerns of pregnancy and contraception may say that they enjoy sex more than ever. This includes a substantial number of American women who have had a hysterectomy. However, in cultures where sexuality is only valued as long as reproduction is possible, the loss of libido and the perception of painful intercourse is unfortunately very common. In Nigeria, for instance, 70 percent of women report being totally abstinent even before they pass their first decade beyond menopause. Their male partners generally take new wives with whom they can have more children. Not long after this, these women experience a loss of desire and other negative feelings concerning sex which cannot be coincidental.

Thus, again it's very vital to consider and confront how you and your partner might feel about your sexuality after a hysterectomy. Instead of dismissing or ignoring any negative feelings, come to terms with them before having a hysterectomy or, better yet, don't have it done!

Does all of this mean that if a woman experiences sexual dysfunction after a hysterectomy that it's all in her mind? Not by a long shot. As we've already discussed, decreased estrogen causes physical changes in the genitalia, including a shortened, less elastic, and drier vagina. The surgery may also alter the vagina because of the formation of scar tissue, or because it has been shortened or tightened. Furthermore, many women say that during an orgasm, their uterus contracts causing pleasurable sensations. Obviously, if a uterus is no longer present, it cannot contribute to orgasm. Likewise, the absence of the cervix may change a woman's sensation during intercourse and may contribute to painful sex because the cervix (being absent) can no longer produce lubrication when a woman becomes aroused. Finally, removal of the ovaries removes one important source of testosterone—the hormone believed to play the greatest role in sex drive. The surgery results in immediate discomfort, of course, but of greater concern are permanent changes in a woman's pelvic anatomy that may be a life-long consequence resulting in life-long sexual problems.

Unfortunately, there may not be easy solutions to these physical changes. A gynecologist may brush them off, and say that artificial hormones or lubricating jellies will compensate. While there is no disputing that they can be helpful, they are *no substitute.* As author Susanne Morgan, who herself has had a hysterectomy, points out, lubricating jellies restore wetness to the vagina, but they do nothing to replace the lack of arousal that would have stimulated the vagina to become lubricated in the first place. As far as hormone replacement therapy is concerned, she also makes an important point:

> Articles implying that estrogen replacement makes everything exactly
> as before are misleading. No one tries to convince a diabetic that the

insulin shots are exactly the same as the insulin produced naturally in the body. A diabetic knows that he or she must take care not to get out of balance and that the insulin simply moderates some of the changes. Even if menopause were an "estrogen deficiency disease" as some people try to portray it, taking estrogen could not totally prevent all changes or adjustments.

So again, don't have a hysterectomy unless you are convinced that there is no other solution to your problem. And don't expect (even if you are told to the contrary) that you will feel exactly the same as before. You may feel the same; you may feel better; or you may feel worse. While we've already said there are no miraculous solutions to sexual dysfunction, the following are some suggestions.

Staying "Sexy"

Sex therapists Masters and Johnson (among others) believe that sexually active women avoid the "atrophic changes" normally caused by a decline in estrogen. No one is sure why this "use it or lose it" phenomenon occurs, although a couple of theories were put forth earlier in this chapter.

In addition, hormone replacement is helpful as mentioned earlier. Estrogen restores vaginal tone and lubrication. Progesterone may decrease depression (which would thus enhance sexual interest). And testosterone increases libido, although it must be given judiciously because of its negative side effects.

A water-based lubricant, such as K-Y Jelly, can provide artificial moisture in the vagina that will decrease painful penetration. While this doesn't substitute for natural arousal, by preventing pain, it may stimulate your body's own natural processes by promoting relaxation and enjoyment.

Finally, to help a woman to cope with purely psychological barriers to sexual enjoyment following a hysterectomy or menopause, a number of books and other resources are available on the subject. (See Appendix A for a listing of some of these resources.) Most of all, remember that stating sexy is a state of mind that needs to be nourished by spontaneous emotion and experimentation.

Choosing a Therapist: A Self-Help Guide

Many women and their families may desire and benefit from some form of counseling or psychotherapy when faced with the issue of hysterectomy. However, you may be unsure of how to locate one that suits your needs best. The following are some "commonsense" tips to help guide you.

1. *Check credentials.* There are myriad titles and levels of training to sift through when trying to find an appropriate match for your particular wants and needs. The following are the commonly used titles and their definition:

   - *Psychotherapist.* A "psychotherapist" may imply any level of training drawn from a variety of backgrounds. There are no laws governing who may use this title; it is a self-imposed label. Therefore, a psychotherapist may be a psychiatric nurse specialist, a social worker—even someone with a college degree in psychology. While it's most important that the individual you consult has experience in your problem and that you feel comfortable with him, this is a case of *caveat emptor* (let the buyer beware). Be sure that your so-called psychotherapist has the proper training and qualifications.

   - *Psychologist.* Anyone using the title psychologist must have a doctoral degree (PhD). These individuals undergo approximately five years of postgraduate work and their specialty is "talk therapy." There are two types of psychologists who have equal levels of training, but with a differing focus. A "clinical psychologist" has the title, "PsyD." Their training emphasizes more clinical experience versus the traditional "PhD" whose training is split between clinical aspects and academic research.

   - *Psychiatrist.* A psychiatrist is a physician (MD) specializing in emotional illness. He has gone through medical school and done a residency in psychiatry. Unlike other types of therapists, he is the only one licensed to prescribe and dispense medications (except for, in some states, psychiatric nurse practitioners). Therefore, if you require antidepressants or perhaps hormones (some psychiatrists would prefer to leave that to your gynecologist), they are a good choice.

     Remember, too, that a reputable pyschotherapist or psychologist who determines that your problem requires medication will refer you to a psychiatrist with whom he collaborates. You can then continue to see your nonphysician provider for talk therapy and the doctor for medication.

2. *Consider cost.* Psychotherapy can be a costly undertaking which is not always covered by medical insurance plans. If this is the case for you, it's worth looking into community mental health centers or teaching clinics

affiliated with major universities that have doctoral programs in clinical psychology. The latter utilize students who are *supervised* by advisors in the therapy they provide. Both resources usually offer low-cost counseling or have a sliding fee scale based on your ability to pay.

3. *Get referrals from reliable friends and colleagues.* They may be a good lead and starting point—one preferable to the yellow pages. Just remember that a therapist may consider that there is a conflict of interest if he is also seeing your friend. However, even if you can't be taken on as a client by this therapist, he can refer you to someone else. It's a good "networking" move.

4. *Shop around.* Call to make an appointment with one or more therapists that you are considering. Honestly explain that you wish to have a trial session with them to see if they can help you with your problem. In the trial session, *go with your gut feeling* about this person. Consider the following:

   - *Do you feel at ease with this person?* Of course, there is always a certain amount of unease. After all, this is your first interaction with a stranger with whom you will be sharing the intimate feelings and details of your life. However, a good therapist will recognize this, and should be able to put you at ease.

   - *Is the therapist talking too much?* In the first one or two sessions, *you* should be doing the bulk of the talking. Early on, it is the role of the therapist to be the *interviewer.* He or she should be eliciting information about you and the details of the problem by *asking questions.* It is too soon for them to be analyzing the situation, drawing conclusions and advising you on major life changes. Beware if they are talking more than they are listening.

   - *Do you feel as though this person really "hears" you?* In other words, does the therapist seem to understand and empathize? You should feel that a strong alliance is possible with this individual—that they will be helpful and trustworthy.

   - *Do you perceive that the two of you have the same or similar value systems?* This is especially important when choosing a sex therapist. You have to feel that the therapist is not being judgmental so that you can be totally open and honest.

   - *What is the therapist's clinical orientation or vision of psychotherapy?* In other words, does the therapist's mode of treatment involve a long-term commitment (e.g., an analytic approach) or do they subscribe to a more short-term model of therapy? Does the type of practice they have fit in with the type of problem you need help with? For example, someone who wants to quit smoking would be better off with a behavioral therapist than he would be engaging in years of psychoanalysis!

5. *Consider a female therapist.* For some women, because of the nature of the problem, having another woman to talk to is essential; for others it is not. Go with what feels right *to you.*

6. *Ask the therapist if he or she has any experience with menopause- or hysterectomy-related problems.*

7. *Once in therapy, evaluate the following:*

   • *Are you making progress?* Remember that change doesn't happen overnight, but you should get a sense that things are moving forward. If they are not, honestly consider whether it's because of you or because of the therapist. Don't hesitate to *bring it up* in your sessions—this may certainly change the pace of things.

   • *Is the therapist acting inappropriately?* If you feel that a therapist's behavior is somehow improper (especially a sex therapist's behavior), discontinue seeing that therapist and consider whether you need to report him to the proper authorities.

8. *Remember that therapy and therapists are not "forever."* If you feel you have made a mistake in choosing someone, you can always make a change.

Summary

The onset of menopause, for some women, may be associated with noticeable changes in the functioning of their bodies. This is especially true for those women whose menopause is sudden and dramatic due to the removal or their uterus and ovaries.

The universal changes that occur, of course, include the end of menstruation and the ability to bear children. For some women, this marks the beginning of a new era of sexual freedom and the pursuit of a new lifestyle that might mean, for example, embarking on a career unencumbered by family responsibilities. Other women, especially those whose personal satisfaction and self-esteem are intimately linked with motherhood, may experience some depression with the loss of these functions.

Women undergoing menopause may also notice a range of other effects, including hot flushes or changes in their skin and sexual organs, to name a few. No two women experience menopause in the same way. It's important to recognize that you may not have any or all of these symptoms and that many of the symptoms are transient as your body adjusts. Frequently, menopausal symptoms may be ameliorated—even eliminated—by hormone replacement therapy. Today, this is safer and more convenient than ever. In addition, it seems to safeguard against osteoporosis and heart disease—two enemies of the older woman.

This does *not* mean that a woman should consider hysterectomy, except as a last resort, because the effects of "instant menopause" are significant, and cannot be fully compensated for by ERT. In addition, the younger a woman is at the time of her surgery, the more likely she is to fall victim to a host of problems, including psychological ones. Hysterectomies on young women for benign diseases result in the highest rates of depression.

In Chapter Nine, we address some of controversies and concerns women face if hysterectomy is inevitable.

9

Damage Control: When
Hysterectomy Is Unavoidable

Excluding the effects of oophorectomy, the results of hysterectomy are extraordinarily good. . . . What then of the many women who, after a hysterectomy, are left chronic invalids or full of complaints? . . . These women suffered the same type of symptoms previously, or at any rate they are of the complaining type with a background of emotional disturbance. Often they are fussy, continuously demanding attention and sympathy from a husband who is perhaps too considerate. The very idea of "having the womb removed" surrounds them with an aura of mystery and fragility to the unknowing and unsuspecting male . . . it should always be explained clearly that hysterectomy by itself should have no physical effect except to cause amenorrhoea (lack of menses), and should not materially affect a woman's way of life, sexual or otherwise.

—Sir Norman Jeffcoate
Jeffcoates' Principles of Gynaecology, 1987 Edition

Up to now, we have spent considerable time discussing the reasons to avoid having a hysterectomy as well as the latest alternative treatments available. However, we have also seen that there are still rare occasions when having a hysterectomy is the best, perhaps the only choice. This chapter addresses three questions of vital importance to women who are faced with the inevitable hysterectomy.

- What type of hysterectomy should I have?

- Should I keep my ovaries?

- Is hormone replacement therapy after hysterectomy in my best interest?

Understanding the Hysterectomy Procedure

There are so many variants to the hysterectomy procedure that it's important here to define and clarify each. If your gynecologist recommends a hysterectomy, be sure that you understand exactly what he means by this and exactly how extensive the surgery will be. In addition, you'll want to know by what route the uterus will be removed and if the ovaries are to remain intact. Hysterectomies are performed two ways. An incision may be made in the abdomen or within the vagina. There are different indications for these two routes and advantages and disadvantages to both. We'll discuss this at greater length later in the chapter. To begin, let us summarize the various types of hysterectomies, both abdominal and vaginal. (It may be helpful to refer to the accompanying diagrams shown in Figure 9.1.)

The Partial or Subtotal Hysterectomy

During this procedure, the entire body of the uterus is removed, but the cervix is left intact.

The Complete or Total Abdominal Hysterectomy (TAH)

In this case, the entire uterus, including the cervix, is removed but all other pelvic structures remain.

The Total Abdominal Hysterectomy with Bilateral Salpingo-Oophorectomy (TAH-BSO)

Here, both ovaries and fallopian tubes are removed along with the uterus.

The Radical Hysterectomy

This operation is generally reserved for cancerous conditions and involves removal of the uterus, ovaries, fallopian tubes, the upper portions of the vagina, and the pelvic lymph nodes.

The Vaginal Hysterectomy

This operation involves making an incision in the upper portion of the vagina and removing the uterus through it. Generally, only the uterus and cervix are excised in this manner although it is technically possible for an experienced surgeon to also remove the ovaries via this route.

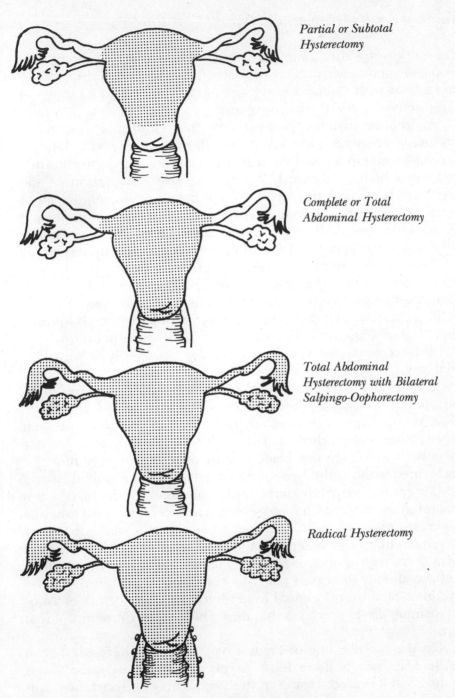

Partial or Subtotal Hysterectomy

Complete or Total Abdominal Hysterectomy

Total Abdominal Hysterectomy with Bilateral Salpingo-Oophorectomy

Radical Hysterectomy

Figure 9.1   Variations of the hysterectomy procedure.

Vaginal versus Abdominal: "Womb" for Choice

In some cases, either a vaginal or an abdominal hysterectomy may be performed to accomplish the same goal. Thus it's important to be familiar with the pros and cons of each approach so that you can discuss them with your surgeon.

Abdominal hysterectomies are the "tried and true" approach. An incision may be made longitudinally or crosswise—the latter is generally lower in the abdomen and may allow a woman to continue to wear a bikini afterward. When extensive exploration of the abdomen is needed and/or when it is necessary to remove all of the pelvic organs, abdominal hysterectomy is necessary because it allows the surgeon a thorough view of the pelvic cavity. For instance, if a woman has cancer or if she and her physician feel hysterectomy is absolutely necessary in a case of severe, recurrent pelvic inflammatory disease or large fibroids causing significant pelvic pain, it should be performed abdominally. In fact, in any case of massive pelvic adhesions or other severe pelvic pathology, the abdominal approach is suggested. Unfortunately, both the operation itself and the recovery period are generally longer, as will be your hospital stay.

If your doctor tells you that he can "get your uterus out in 30 minutes," *you should seriously consider why it is being removed in the first place.* Vaginal hysterectomies are indeed quicker operations, but they require a great deal of skill. This is because there is greater potential to damage the bladder and rectum and they must be performed without the benefit of a view of the abdominal cavity.

Generally, vaginal hysterectomies are best performed for a prolapsed uterus (see Chapter Seven). However, sometimes vaginal hysterectomies are also carried out to eradicate a small fibroid or for recurrent uterine bleeding. *A vaginal hysterectomy that is suggested for these two reasons alone can probably be avoided,* using the methods we have already discussed (such as endometrial ablation). Therefore, the "30 minute" vaginal hysterectomies that doctors boast of performing are procedures that don't have to be done in the first place!

On the positive side of vaginal hysterectomy, there will be no visible scar (nor is there likely to be adhesion formation), and healing will be rapid. However, the vagina may be shortened during the procedure, potentially exacerbating any postmenopausal sexual problems.

Speeding Your Recovery

In either case, it's important to have a frank discussion with your practitioner regarding what to expect during the recovery period. Immediately after the surgery, and no matter how uncomfortable you may feel, you should try to walk with assistance. Remaining stationary retards circulation and increases your risk of developing a *thrombophlebitis* or blood clot in your leg. In addition, you should follow the coughing and deep breathing instructions you will no doubt be taught by a nurse. Both of these steps decrease the likelihood of your developing pneumonia after the surgery. (Lying immobile in bed allows fluid to accumulate in the lungs. This serves as a perfect incubating medium for bacteria and hence, pneumonia may result).

Because of the economics of health care, people are being discharged from hospitals much sooner postoperatively than in the past. It's important to recognize that being sent home doesn't mean you are ready to resume your former role of "superwoman." Remember you may need to be on pain medications and these can affect your judgment. Arrange for someone to take care of you (and your children, if they are young), for as long as possible. Avoid lifting heavy loads, moving large objects, doing major housework, and driving for as long as your doctor tells you is necessary. Again, discuss with your doctor when you can resume working, having sex, douching, and particpating in very active sports. Expect that it may be two or more months before you can again be fully functional. Be sure to contact your physician if you develop a fever, worsening pain, significant bleeding, or discharge from the wound.

Being an Advocate: Keeping Your Ovaries

One should never forget that ovarian cancer is a very serious disease, difficult to detect, difficult to manage, and ultimately deadly for 1 in every 100 women. No doubt this is what has prompted surgeons to remove innumerable ovaries through the years. However, one should also never forget that there was also a time when nymphomania was considered a serious disease, and zealous surgeons literally used to display their prized ovaries on silver platters to the awe and rapturous applause of their colleagues at medical conventions.

According to the American College of Obstetricians and Gynecologists, *an estimated 700 prophylactic oophorectomies would be required to prevent a single case of ovarian cancer!* And, in light of what we know can be the sometimes dramatic and debilitating effects associated with "instant menopause" (see Chapter Eight), it is in the best interest of every woman and her doctor to carefully weigh the pros and cons. As one example, a premenopausal woman undergoing hysterectomy and oophorectomy has three times the risk of developing coronary artery disease and thus is much more likely to die of a heart condition than from *any* form of cancer, ovarian or otherwise.

Even more troubling, there have been reports in the scientific literature of women developing cancer identical to ovarian cancer years after bilateral oophorectomy! Doctors still don't understand this phenomenon, although it may be related to ovarian cancer being able to develop in abdominal tissue that was a precursor to ovary formation in the embryo. Thus, removing a woman's ovaries is not a 100 percent guarantee that she will never develop ovarian cancer.

If a woman is to have her ovaries removed, she should probably undergo hormone replacement therapy to minimize the side effects discussed in Chapter Eight, especially osteoporosis and cardiovascular disease. Yet, as we shall see, this is a major decision with some disadvantages and some risks. Furthermore, not every woman is willing or able to take hormonal supplements for what may be the rest of her life. Finally, ERT does not solve all of the potential and troublesome side effects (i.e., skin changes and decreased sexual desire) because it cannot substitute for what nature provides. Consider this statement by the American College of Obstetricians and Gynecologists:

> Hormonal replacement with estrogen and a progestogen [progesterone] is not physiologic. In premenopausal women who have undergone oophorectomy, gonadotrophin [sex hormone] levels do not return to premenopausal levels following estrogen-progestogen therapy, indicating that feedback control on the hypothalamic-pituitary axis [nervous system] is incompletely mimicked by these two exogenous hormones.

Some surgeons try to convince women to have their ovaries removed at the time of hysterectomy to prevent them from needing another operation in the future. For most women, this will *never* be necessary. The incidence of repeat operations for removal of residual ovaries is anywhere from less than 1 to 5 percent. Looked at from another angle, of all the women with ovarian cancer, few have had a prior hysterectomy. (Estimates vary widely, from less than 1 percent to no more than 14 percent.)

There are some criteria that you should consider when deciding whether or not to preserve your ovaries. Your age is important. Ovarian cancer is extremely rare before the age of 40 and menopause is not likely to occur for a number of years. Therefore, don't let anyone talk you into a prophylactic oophorectomy before your fortieth birthday. However, it may be reasonable to have an oophorectomy after age 50. In offering my opinion, I may *advise* a woman to do so. However, in such matters when it's not a life and death decision, but more a consideration of *how a woman may feel* faced with the loss of her ovaries (she is now castrated), I firmly believe that it is the role of the gynecologist to advise, inform, and guide a woman in her decision—*not to make the decision for her.* It is she who is going to have to live with the consequences and with her feelings afterward, therefore it is she who must make the ultimate choice after informed and thoughtful consideration.

Besides age, there are other factors that may tip the balance either in favor of or against this procedure. Oophorectomy may make sense depending on your personal or family medical history. For example, if you have had ovarian cysts in the past or endometriosis, you may find that pain may recur or persist after your hysterectomy, necessitating oophorectomy. If you have had breast, endometrial, or colon cancer, you are at increased risk for ovarian cancer and should consider prophylactic oophorectomy. Likewise, having close relatives with breast or ovarian cancer increases your risk. Conversely, situations that have allowed the ovary to "rest" for a while, such as having had children or having taken birth control pills (even for as short a time as three months) statistically decreases ovarian cancer risk and should be taken into consideration.

All in all, it is a complex decision that requires a woman to weigh her risks against her willingness to weather the menopausal "storm," which can be expected to be more severe when induced surgically.

Hormone Replacement: Consider It Carefully

The development of hormone supplements to curb the deleterious effects of menopause has proven to be a tremendous advance in women's health care. They are relatively safe (not seeming to share some of the worrisome side effects of their distant relative—birth control pills). They are also becoming more convenient, as they are now available as creams, suppositories, and transdermal patches as well as in their traditional forms: tablets and injections. (Note: The patches are placed on the skin and the medication slowly releases in a controlled dosage over several days. They seem to bypass the liver when they are being processed by the body, and therefore may have less side effects. However, for this reason, they may not be as effective for all postmenopausal indications.)

However, despite safety, efficacy, and improved convenience, ERT remains controversial (see Table 9.1).

Table 9.1   Hormone replacement therapy: Should you or shouldn't you?

Hormone	Advantages	Disadvantages
Estrogen	Relieves hot flashes and flushes.	May have unpleasant side effects, such as breast tenderness, weight gain, nausea, headaches.
	May help with bladder dysfunction and discomforts.	
	Reverses aging effects on vagina.	May cause high blood pressure (dose related).
	Prevents osteoporosis.	If taken without progesterone, carries increased risk of endometrial cancer.
	May prevent heart disease by altering cholesterol.	
	May help with insomnia, especially if due to nocturnal flushes.	May increase risk of gallbladder disease.

(continued)

Table 9.1 Hormone replacement therapy (continued)

Hormone	Advantages	Disadvantages
	May help with emotional state, depending on underlying causes and other life events.	May increase chance of breast cancer; extremely controversial.
	May help sex life, especially if problems are related to vaginal discomforts.	
Progesterone	Seems to negate endometrial cancer risk for women on ERT.	May cause vaginal bleeding, weight gain or increased appetite, mood swings, breast tenderness or acne (temporary phenomena).
	May prevent breast cancer; extremely controversial.	
		May eliminate benefits of ERT on the heart due to increase in LDL cholesterol.
Testosterone	Generally increases libido.*	May cause masculinizing side effects, such as growth of facial hair, lowering of vocal register, and acne.
	May help reduce hot flashes.	

*Unlike estrogen, which mainly seems to aid in sexual dysfunction by increasing vaginal lubrication and preventing atrophic vaginitis, testosterone seems to increase sexual arousal and the number of orgasms achieved.

Endometrial Cancer Risk

In the mid-1970s, two highly regarded studies were published in the prestigious *New England Journal of Medicine* citing a substantially increased risk of endometrial cancer associated with estrogen use. To make matters worse, these frightening results were confirmed in the numerous investigations that followed, sometimes revealing as much as an eightfold increase in risk—a risk that did not go away even if a woman stopped taking estrogen. In short order, the "fountain of youth" had turned into a "dance with death." Doctors stopped prescribing estrogen and women stopped taking it.

In subsequent years, further work determined that so-called unopposed estrogen was at the root of the danger. This was because constant exposure of the uterus to estrogen, as in the case of naturally occurring hormonal imbalance and dysfunctional uterine bleeding, leads to endometrial hyperplasia. Hyperplasia may lead to cancer.

It was determined that if, as in the premenopausal state, a woman was given progesterone in addition to estrogen, this abnormal buildup of the uterine lining would be circumvented. Today, estrogen replacement therapy has regained its good name, but it is *highly recommended* that it be cycled with a progesterone in women who still have their uterus.

Of course, progesterone is not without *its* price. Depending on the type of progesterone you take, there may be a negating of the cardioprotective effects of estrogen. Specifically, progesterone increases LDL cholesterol. Therefore, it's important that you take a type of progesterone least likely to have this effect, *and* that you take it long enough to protect against cancer (at least 7 to 10 days each month).

Finally, be prepared for the fact that estrogen with progesterone may again make you feel as you did when you were menstruating. There may be a return of acne, breast tenderness, mood swings, and, perhaps most inconvenient of all, vaginal bleeding. However, some of these side effects may be ameliorated by adjusting the dosage of the progesterone. More important, many women consider all of this worthwhile to protect themselves against osteoporosis, cardiac disease, and endometrial cancer.

Breast Cancer Risk

In 1988, doctors at the Mayo Clinic very effectively summarized the available information on hormone replacement therapy and the risk of breast cancer. They stated:

> Methodologic deficiencies and inconsistencies have prevented a clear understanding of whether estrogen replacement therapy increases the risk of breast cancer. Some investigators have shown that a slight but statistically insignificant increased risk of breast cancer is associated with the oral use of estrogens. Others have concluded that estrogens do not increase the risk of breast cancer and may improve the prognosis in those in whom breast cancer does develop during estrogen therapy. In any event, the risk seems to be small and has not been found consistently. . . .

Believe it or not, this statement doesn't begin to highlight all of the confusion and controversy surrounding this particular issue. The following are some of the unanswered questions.

Is dosage and duration of therapy important? Some researchers believe that how much estrogen you take and for how long is at the root of the question. One large study found long-term use in moderately high doses could be linked to breast cancer whereas short-term, low-dose therapy could not.

How about the way in which you take the estrogen? A group of investigators in North Carolina revealed that the risk of breast cancer with oral forms was neglible, but that injectable estrogen increased risk four times over. However, lest you gain a false sense of security from pill use, a study of over 23,000 Swedish women published in a 1989 issue of the *New England Journal of Medicine* seems to indicate that not all oral estrogens may be created equal. That is, the type of oral estrogen you take may make the difference between no risk and nearly *double* the risk of breast cancer. (Fortunately, the safest estrogen pills are also those most commonly prescribed in the United States. Specifically, synthetic so-called estradiol-type estrogens were implicated while natural estrogens were not.)

Can progesterone safeguard against any increased risk of breast cancer? A 1986 editorial appearing in *Obstetrics and Gynecology* seemed at first to support this view, citing the evidence of two well-publicized studies by Dr. Gambrell and his colleagues. However, claiming that these investigations had "serious methodologic flaws," the editors concluded:

> Current evidence does not justify the practice of adding progestin to postmenopausal estrogen therapy in an attempt to reduce the risk of breast cancer.

Do women with benign breast disease (i.e., "cystic breasts") add to their risk of developing cancer if they take ERT? Likewise, what about women who have had their ovaries removed? Again, it depends on which scientific study you believe. Some say taking ERT reduces breast cancer risk; others directly contradict them! In one study of Australian women, breast cancer risk reduction in both of these areas was dramatic: 40 percent for women with benign breast disease; 70 percent for women with bilateral oophorectomy. In another study, by British physicians, "[The] most consistently identified [risk factor for breast cancer] has been a history of benign breast disease." Furthermore, these same doctors found that "Although hormone use was not associated with any substantial overall risk, there was some hazard suggested among women who have received hormones following bilateral oophorectomy."

Another sketchy area is whether it's advisable to commence ERT if there is a family history of breast cancer. Dr. Wingo and her colleagues found a "twofold increased risk" if women had a close relative who had breast cancer.

The most frustrating aspect to this, of course, is that we as doctors cannot provide ourselves or our patients with concrete and consistent information. Clearly, additional work needs to be done. We need to discover whether women will exhibit the increased incidence of breast cancer found when laboratory animals are given ERT. We must resolve whether estrogen supplementation will increase breast cancer risk in the same manner as do conditions that naturally increase estrogen exposure, such as obesity, infrequent or late pregnancies, and hormonal imbalance, to name a few. Finally, we must face the fact that all of the data—pro and con—must be tempered by time. That is, cancer often takes many

Hysterectomy: A Self-Help Guide

If your doctor suggests hysterectomy, *proceed with caution!*

First find out . . .

WHO . . . is this doctor? Is he someone you know and trust? Does he have a good reputation in the community and are his credentials beyond reproach? Even so, get a second—even a third—opinion before consenting to surgery.

WHAT . . . does he intend to take out? Believe it or not, in talking to women who have had hysterectomies, some do not know *exactly what was removed!* Remember all the variations and permutations of hysterectomy, and make sure you understand clearly if only your uterus is to be removed. If so, is it your entire uterus or will the cervix be left behind? Will the ovaries, fallopian tubes, lymph nodes, portions of the vagina, appendix, or other tissues also be taken out? If so, why? If not, why not? *Make sure that you are especially clear about and comfortable with the discussion concerning the removal of your ovaries.* Try to have a say in the matter when there is a choice and consider all the pros and cons in your case.

WHEN . . . does the surgery need to be done? Postpone scheduling the operation if it is not clearly an emergency. (Most of the time, it is not.) Allow yourself time to seek other opinions, to carefully consider what the loss of your uterus will mean to you and your spouse, and to adjust to the idea if you elect to proceed with hysterectomy. Women who did this had significantly less psychological problems afterward than those who rushed ahead.

WHERE . . . will the incision be made? Do you have a choice of a vaginal versus an abdominal hysterectomy? For extensive pelvic disease, you want to campaign for an abdominal procedure whereas vaginal hysterectomies are preferred for prolapse. (If a vaginal hysterectomy is not being performed for a prolapse, *chances are it doesn't have to be done at all!*) Don't try to talk a surgeon who is comfortable with abdominal hysterectomies into doing a vaginal one for you or vice versa. Instead, find a doctor who is an expert at the procedure you desire.

WHY . . . do you need this hysterectomy? Last but not least, remember that the best "damage control" for hysterectomies is obviously *avoiding* them! Now that you have read this book, you know that the so-called indications for hysterectomies do not mean that they are truly "necessary." There may be alternative treatments, and there may be time to "watch and wait." *Don't let anyone*—not even a renowned physician with a lot of impressive degrees and credentials—*talk you into a hysterectomy* if you feel uncomfortable with the idea. Carefully consider the options. *Remember what is done cannot be undone.*

years to show itself. For example, workers exposed to asbestos as young men did not begin to reveal exorbitant rates of lung cancer for 20 to 30 years.

For now, the best we can do is act with caution. It's probably not a good idea to take ERT if you already have a risk factor for breast cancer. In addition, special attention should be devoted to regular, thorough breast self-examinations and to having mammograms according to the recommended guidelines for women over age 35. This advice applies whether or not you ultimately decide to take estrogen.

Incidentally, cervical cancer and ovarian cancer do not appear to be affected by hormone replacement therapy.

Other Risks

Many of the official contraindications to ERT are based on some of the problems that have been known to develop when women have been on birth control pills. As we've already mentioned, oral contraceptives differ fundamentally in type and dosage from post-menopausal hormone supplements. Nevertheless, until research-ers know more, it is best to err on the safe side. Therefore, since estrogen is processed by the liver, ERT is not advised for women with either liver or gallbladder disease. In addition, because it may affect blood clotting, estrogen should be avoided if you have had a blot clot form in your leg (phlebitis) or if one has blocked off the blood supply to your heart or brain resulting, respectively, in either a heart attack or a stroke. Have your blood pressure and cholesterol checked before embarking on ERT to avoid any contribution to arteriosclerotic heart disease. Finally, certain preexisting medical conditions may worsen with ERT and thus require careful watching. For example: migraine headaches, endometriosis, and fibroids.

Summary

To minimize the damage that may be done when hysterectomy cannot be avoided, it's important to consider several factors. They include whether you can choose the type of hysterectomy you have, and whether you can safely preserve your ovaries to avoid making an undesirable situation worse.

Certainly, if you have this surgery, you should consider the relative advantages and disadvantages to hormonal replacement therapy in your case. No set rules and regulations apply. On the positive side, as discussed at length in Chapter Eight, ERT can help to reverse such unpleasant side effects as: hot flushes, atrophic vaginitis, bladder discomfort, and perhaps even depression and sexual difficulties. More important, it will most likely impact on your risk for osteoporosis and arteriosclerosis—both deadly diseases.

However, you may be exposing yourself to a greater risk of breast cancer and possibly other serious medical conditions, such as thrombophlebitis. (Remember, the incidence of thrombophlebitis is a lot lower with ERT than with oral contraceptives.) Furthermore, ERT requires years of compliance with taking medications that may cause unpleasant side effects. This is an inconvenience many women find unacceptable.

Women on hormonal replacement must insist on the lowest effective dose, and should discuss with their doctors whether less invasive routes, such as transdermal patches, will be effective in accomplishing whatever their goal was in commencing ERT. They must be diligent when it comes to following through with screening tests to monitor their health while on ERT. These include: regular blood pressure readings, blood tests for cholesterol levels, breast and pelvic exams (including mammograms, PAP smears, and periodic endometrial biopsies, as needed). Yearly endometrial biopsies are important because they will assure you and your physician that hyperplasia is not present.

The rewards of hormone replacement therapy may be a longer, more productive life! Consider this statement by Drs. Hillner, Hollenberg, and Pauker, which was published in the *American Journal of Medicine* in 1986:

> . . . estrogen therapy provides a significant gain in quality-adjusted life expectancy. In considering the efficacy of any drug, all the benefits of the drug as well as all its risks must be included. If the beneficial effect of estrogens on cardiovascular mortality is confirmed, it will overshadow all other effects. Any recommendation about postmenopausal estrogens with respect to osteoporosis that excludes their cardiovascular effects markedly underestimates the potential gains from therapy.

Dr. Elizabeth Barrett-Conner adds:

For the average North American woman, who will be postmenopausal for one third of her life, the benefits of estrogen seem strongly established. In addition to its unequivocal value for the relief of menopausal symptoms, the long-term use of postmenopausal estrogen can prevent osteoporosis and its debilitating or fatal consequences. The use of estrogen must also be considered in light of a possible 50 percent reduction in the risk of cardiovascular disease and the possibility of a nearly doubled risk of breast cancer. In this decade the increased risk of endometrial cancer associated with estrogen use led to the frequent addition of a progestin to estrogen-replacement therapy, which further complicates the tallying of risks and benefits.

Up to now, we've examined all of the options for both avoiding hysterectomy whenever possible, and for maintaining damage control, when hysterectomy is unavoidable. We've discussed what you might expect to experience in the aftermath of hysterectomy as well as how to handle the effects. *Now it's up to you!*

Epilogue

Future Hopes

Women truthfully are unique mammals, carrying, feeding, and nurturing their young; surviving a greater percentage of the time in utero and earlier in the neonatal period and, ultimately, living longer than men.

—Derek Llewellyn-Jones, 1971

I'd like to end this book on a hopeful note. Much of what has been explored here pointed to a past history which was not always encouraging. Thus what was said was not always positive. Sometimes it was downright critical. However, this book is being published at the onset of a new decade when the future is bright and promising for women suffering from a variety of conditions that at one time would have mandated hysterectomy.

In 1900, Dr. George Engelmann spoke before a meeting of the American Gynecological Society. This forward-thinking man's words could not have rung any truer then than they do today. He said:

> We seem to have attained the apex of surgical achievement but there are peaks beyond, new fields to conquer. . . . We cannot safely rest on past achievements; we must struggle onward. . . . Along the lines of extirpation, we can no longer advance; we must look to preservation, to the conserving of the function, and this I believe to be the surgery of the twentieth century.

In order to fulfill the aspirations so eloquently stated by Dr. Engelmann, much work still needs to be done. In writing this book, I hope to educate women about their bodies. Specifically, it is my goal to contribute to raising women's consciousness concerning hysterectomy—a procedure that I believe to be performed far too frequently without knowledge or consideration of the alternatives.

In addition, I hope that physicians will also become more enlightened, emphasizing research and development in the areas of medical versus surgical alternatives to hysterectomy; the utilization of lasers which offer a safer and less invasive option than traditional surgery, and improvements in therapy for all gynecological concerns from cancer to menopause.

Finally, I hope that we will soon see the day when the crisis in health care brought about by a shortage of everything from nurses to dollars will force the medical community and those responsible for administering our health insurance system to recognize that the less-invasive alternatives to hysterectomy are much more cost-effective. For example, while "illness-oriented" health care plans presently cover the cost of a hysterectomy, they do not generally pay for such health maintenance procedures as Pap smears. Yet this simple, inexpensive test has prevented countless numbers of hysterectomies through early cancer detection. Likewise, insurance companies do not reimburse for many laser procedures because they are considered "too new and experimental." However, studies performed by myself and others have proven their safety and efficacy. Moreover, these may frequently be performed as ambulatory surgeries, saving the costs of hospital beds and nursing care, not to mention time lost from work as a result of a shortened recovery period.

I was trained in a big city hospital where a premium was placed on the number of hysterectomies you did and not on how good you were at preserving someone's uterus. We often did not anticipate, nor did we consider, the tremendous impact such surgery would have on a woman's life—on the way in which she and her loved ones might view her once her reproductive capabilities had been taken away from her. The way you are trained stays with you for a while, and old habits die hard. In the seventeenth century, Joseph Addison said, "When men are easy in their circumstances, they are naturally enemies to innovations." However, the time has come for all of us—patients, doctors, health care administrators— to look toward the future. Today, 50 percent of all hysterectomies can be eliminated by critical evaluation; another 40 percent by advanced medical and surgical techniques. We must recognize that alternatives to hysterectomy benefit each and every one of us. The time to change is now.

A

Helpful Organizations

Hysterectomy

Hysterectomy Educational Resources and Services Foundation
(HERS)
422 Bryn Mawr Avenue
Bala Cynwyd, Pennsylvania 19004
215-667-7757

This foundation provides free information on alternative treatments
for hysterectomy as well as on coping with hysterectomy. It publishes a newsletter, sponsors conferences, and offers telephone
counseling. Counseling sessions are conducted by appointment
only, Monday–Friday, 9:30 A.M. to noon (Eastern Standard Time).
You may call for an appointment or additional information at any
time. There is a 24-hour answering service.

Endometriosis/Infertility

Endometriosis Association
8585 North 76th Place
Milwaukee, Wisconsin 53225
414-355-2200

This is a self-help and support group with over 100 chapters that
provides literature, contact lists, and a bimonthly newsletter. They
have a crisis hotline at the above telephone number which may be
reached Monday–Friday, 8 A.M. to 5 P.M. (Central Time).

RESOLVE
5 Water Street
Arlington, Massachusetts 02174
617-643-2424

This organization offers monthly programs, support groups, counseling, medical referrals, and a newsletter to couples struggling with infertility. Counselors answer calls Monday–Thursday, 9 A.M. to noon and then from 1 P.M. to 4 P.M. (Eastern Standard Time).

The American Fertility Society
2140 11th Avenue South, Number 200
Birmingham, Alabama 35205-2800
205-933-8494

This society provides lists of member physicians in your area, a bibliography and printed publications, including booklets concerning both endometriosis and infertility.

Sexuality/Mental Health

The American Association of Sex Educators, Counselors and
    Therapists (AASECT)
435 North Michigan Avenue, Suite 1717
Chicago, Illinois 60611
312-644-0828

This is primarily a professional organization providing certification and continuing education programs for its members. However, it does provide a free listing of member professionals in each state that may then be further evaluated by you.

Sex Information and Education Council of the United States
    (SIECUS)
32 Washington Place, Suite 52
New York, New York 10003
212-673-3850

This organization serves as an advocacy group and clearinghouse of information that includes: an annotated bibliography, publications, lists of organizations providing referrals to qualified sex therapists, and a unique research library and database available to professionals as well as the general public. It is affiliated with New York University.

Cancer/Smoking Cessation

The National Cancer Institute Office of Cancer Communications
National Cancer Institute
National Institutes of Health
Building 31, Room 10A24
Bethesda, Maryland 20892
Toll-free hotline: 1-800-4-CANCER

This is a government agency that provides free information and operates a hotline from 8 A.M. to midnight, Monday–Friday (Eastern Standard Time).

American Cancer Society
1599 Clifton Road, N.E.
Atlanta, Georgia 30329
404-320-3333
Toll-free information: 1-800-ACS-2345

This is a voluntary organization of several thousand local chapters that provides literature on smoking cessation as well as on all aspects of cancer, including: prevention, diagnosis, treatment, dealing with psychosocial issues, and so forth. It's advised to contact the unit in your area for specific programs and literature. In addition, they maintain a toll-free information line which draws on an extensive computer database.

Heart Disease

American Heart Association
7320 Greenville Avenue
Dallas, Texas 75231
214-373-6300

The American Heart Association provides a variety of materials on: heart attacks, strokes, nutrition, exercise, and how to quit smoking. Again, it's best to contact your local affiliate for specific details.

The National Cholesterol Education Program Information Center
4733 Bethesda Avenue, Suite 530
Bethesda, Maryland 20814
301-951-3260

This agency publishes excellent free resource materials concerning high blood cholesterol.

General Women's Health

The Boston Women's Health Book Collective
240A Elm Street
Somerville, Massachusetts 02144
617-625-0271

Mailing address:
P.O. Box 192
West Somerville, MA 02144

This is a public information center that contains national and international publications concerning women's health and other issues pertaining to women.

National Women's Health Network
1325 G Street, N.W.
Washington, D.C. 20003
202-347-1140

A national organization devoted exclusively to women and health, it publishes a newsletter as well as special "news alerts" concerning issues requiring immediate attention. Both are available to members.

B

Diets to Promote Heart and Bone Health

Eating well is particularly important to the postmenopausal woman. The pages that follow will assist you in choosing foods that are high in calcium and low in cholesterol.

Whether dining out or selecting items in the supermarket, follow these general guidelines in conjunction with the food lists on subsequent pages to stay fit and healthy:

- Include three to four servings of calcium-rich foods in your daily diet, avoiding those foods high in fat and cholesterol.

- Prepare foods simply, by baking, broiling, boiling, stewing, or roasting and eliminating or limiting the use of heavy sauces and gravies.

- Cut down on fat, protein, and caffeine as these impair calcium absorption.

- Read food labels carefully as there are no official, government-regulated definitions for words such as "light," "low calorie," or "natural."

- Favor white-meat poultry and fish. When eating red meat, choose lean cuts of beef with all visible fat removed.

- Use yogurt instead of mayonnaise in dressings.

- Increase fiber-rich foods (such as whole-grain breads, raw fruits, vegetables, and beans).

- Generally eat in moderation to obtain a variety of foods and to maintain ideal body weight. Avoid alcohol, tobacco, and caffeine. All of this will go a long way in increasing your odds for a long and healthy life!

Calcium Content in Milligram of Selected Foods

Food	Portion	Calcium Content
Beverages		
Alcoholic		
Beer	12 oz.	20
Eggnog	4 oz.	45
Gin	1 oz.	0
Wine	4 oz.	5–10
Coffee, brewed	12 oz.	trace
Carbonated drinks		
Cola type drinks	12 oz.	0–trace
Ginger ale	12 oz.	trace
Mineral water	8 oz.	33 (varies)
Orange soda	12 oz.	trace
Root beer	12 oz.	trace
Noncola type drink	12 oz.	trace
Noncarbonated drinks		
Apple juice	6 oz.	10
Cranberry juice	6 oz.	10
Fruit punch	6 oz.	12
Punch	8 oz.	20
Orange juice with added calcium	6 oz.	200–300
Tea	8 oz.	trace
Water, drinking	8 oz.	varies
Bread, Grain, Cereal, Pasta Products		
Bagel	1 medium	20
Biscuit, 2″ diameter, average	1	40
Bread, sliced, cracked wheat	1 slice	20
Raisin bread	1 slice	25
Rye	1 slice	25
White, enriched	1 slice	25
Whole wheat	1 slice	25
Cornbread, whole ground meal	1 piece	95
Corn grits, enriched, cooked	1 cup	2
Dry cereal made with ½ cup milk	1 oz.	150–350
Farina made with milk	¾ cup	150
Fettuccine, cheese sauce	2 oz.	40
Flour, self-rising	1 cup	300
Wheat, all purpose	1 cup	20
White, all purpose	1 cup	18–20

Calcium Content in Milligram of Selected Foods

Food	Portion	Calcium Content
Lasagna, cheese	8 oz.	220
Macaroni, baked with cheese	1 cup	360
Canned with cheese	1 cup	199
Cooked	1 cup	15
Frozen, with cheese	1 cup	235
Manicotti, cheese-filled	8.5 oz.	300–550
Muffin, refined flour	1	35–90
Noodles	1 cup	15
Oat bran, made with milk	1 oz.	150
Oatmeal, made with milk	1 oz.	160–170
Pancakes, buckwheat, 4″ diameter	4	230–390
Made with enriched flour	4	150–190
Pizza, cheese, 10″ diameter, ¼″ thick	1 pizza	620
Rice, converted, before cooking	1 cup	59–65
Brown, before cooking	1 cup	60
White, before cooking	1 cup	45
White, cooked	1 cup	15–20
Roll, breakfast, danish	1 roll	20
Refined flour	1 roll	15–30
Whole wheat	1 roll	34–45
Spaghetti, enriched, cooked	1 cup	14
Tomato sauce, cheese	1 cup	80
Stuffing, bread	½ cup	35–45
Tortilla	1	45
Waffles, frozen	2 small	40–90
Made fresh	1 large	180
Chips and Snacks		
Cheese puffs	1 oz.	16
Cheese straws, 5″ long	10 pieces	150
Corn chips	1 oz.	30–40
Potato chips	10 chips	8
Pretzels	10	6
Tortilla chips	1 oz.	35
Tortilla chips, cheese flavored	1 oz.	50
Dairy Products		
Butter	1 Tbsp.	3
Buttermilk, cultured	8 oz.	300
1% lowfat	8 oz.	300

Calcium Content in Milligram of Selected Foods

Food	Portion	Calcium Content
Cheese		
American cheese spread	1 oz.	175
Blue cheese	1 oz.	140
Camembert cheese	1 oz.	30
Cheddar cheese	1 oz.	210
Cheddar cheese, grated	1 cup	845
Colby cheese	1 oz.	200
Cottage cheese, 1% milkfat	8 oz.	140
2% milkfat	8 oz.	150
4% milkfat	8 oz.	214
Creamed	8 oz.	150
Cream cheese	1 oz.	18
Edam cheese	1 oz.	200
Feta cheese	1 oz.	135
Gouda cheese	1 oz.	190
Monterey cheese	1 oz.	200
Parmesan cheese, grated	1 Tbsp.	65
Hard	1 oz.	325
Reduced calorie, low fat cheese	1 oz.	200
Ricotta cheese	1 oz.	110
Roquefort cheese	1 oz.	175
Sliced cheese, American	1 oz.	150–200
Jalapeno	1 oz.	200
Monterey Jack	1 oz.	200
Souffle, cheese	1 cup	191
Swiss cheese	1 oz.	270–300
Chocolate drink	8 oz.	250
Chocolate milk, 1% lowfat	8 oz.	300
Cream, light	½ cup	130
heavy	½ cup	90
Evaporated milk, regular, skim	8 oz.	500–600
Evaporated condensed milk	8 oz.	800
Goat's milk	8 oz.	300
Ice cream, most flavors	1 cup	175–270
Ice cream stick, vanilla, average	1	60
Instant meal drink made with milk	8 oz.	400–500
Milk, cow's milk, calcium-fortified	8 oz.	500
High protein	8 oz.	350
Lactose-reduced	8 oz.	300
Skim	8 oz.	300

Calcium Content in Milligram of Selected Foods

Food	Portion	Calcium Content
Milk (*cont.*)		
2%	8 oz.	300
Whole milk	8 oz.	300
Milkshake, average vanilla	8 oz.	450
Average chocolate	8 oz.	400
Shake mix, average	8 oz.	300
Mousse	½ cup	100
Non-fat dry milk, prepared	8 oz.	300
Puddings, canned, most flavors	5 oz.	100
Cooked, made with milk	½ cup	150–250
Instant	½ cup	150–250
Sugar-free instant	½ cup	150
Pudding on a stick	1	75
Sour cream	1 Tbsp.	14
Welsh Rarebit	1 cup	582
White Sauce, medium	1 cup	288
Yogurt, frozen, high calcium	8 oz.	300
Frozen, most flavors	6 oz.	150
Frozen yogurt stick	2½ oz.	100–150
Nonfat	8 oz.	450
1% milkfat	8 oz.	400
1.5% milkfat	8 oz.	350
Soft frozen yogurt	3 oz.	60
Desserts and Sweets		
Bread pudding	1 cup	280
Cakes, angel food	1 slice	2–40
Chocolate, chocolate icing	1 slice	70
Cupcake with icing	1	23–35
Fruitcake, average	1 slice	10–30
Gingerbread, average	1 piece	60–80
Pound cake	1 slice	6–15
Sponge cake	1 slice	10–25
White, chocolate icing	1 slice	60–90
Yellow, chocolate icing	1 slice	60–80
Candies, caramels	1 oz.	40
Chocolate chips	1 oz.	25
Fudge, plain	1 oz.	20–30
Hard candies	1 oz.	0
Marshmallow, large	1	1

Calcium Content in Milligram of Selected Foods

Food	Portion	Calcium Content
Milk chocolate	1 oz.	65
Peanut brittle	1 oz.	10
Cookies, average size		
Animal cookies	10	14
Brownie	2 large	15
Chocolate	1	10
Chocolate chip	1	8
Fig bars	1	11
Gingersnaps	1	5
Graham crackers	1	6
Oatmeal	1	7–15
Peanut butter	1	5–12
Sugar	1	6
Custard, homemade with milk, eggs	½ cup	145
Coconut	½ cup	140
Doughnuts, cake type	1	6–25
Gelatin, made with water	1 cup	0
Honey	2 oz.	2–4
Ice cream—see *Dairy Products*		
Ices, flavored	1 cup	0
Jams, preserves	1 Tbsp.	4
Jellies	1 Tbsp.	1–4
Molasses, blackstrap	1 Tbsp.	135
Cane, refined	1 Tbsp.	30–60
Pie, ⅛ of 9" diameter pie		
Apple	1 slice	10
Banana cream	1 slice	130
Butterscotch	1 slice	86
Cherry	1 slice	15–20
Custard	1 slice	70–150
Lemon meringue	1 slice	14–24
Mincemeat	1 slice	20–45
Pumpkin	1 slice	45–95
Puddings—see *Dairy Products*		
Sherbet	1 cup	95
Sugar, brown, dark	1 cup	165
Granulated	1 cup	0–trace
Syrup, maple	2 Tbsp.	40–60
Table blends	2 Tbsp.	18
Tapioca cream pudding	1 cup	170–250

Calcium Content in Milligram of Selected Foods

Food	Portion	Calcium Content
Eggs		
Boiled egg	1 large	28
Egg substitute, average	4 oz.	25–75
Egg substitute with cheese	4 oz.	28–78
Fish and Seafoods		
Clams, steamed or canned	8 oz.	121
Cod, broiled	1 steak	64
Crabmeat, cooked	1 cup	65
Flounder, baked	1 oz.	7
Haddock, fried	3 oz.	11–40
Herring, kippered	1 small	13–45
Lobster, steamed	1 pound	300
Oysters, raw, 13–19 medium	1 cup	226
Salmon, canned	3 oz.	160–250
Red with bones	3.5 oz.	195–350
Sardines, canned with bones	8 medium	350–450
Scallops, breaded, fried	3.5 oz.	110
Shad, baked	1 oz.	7
Shrimp, steamed	3 oz.	95
Swordfish, broiled	1 steak	37
Tuna, canned	3 oz.	6
Clam chowder	1 cup	37–170
Fritters	1 fritter	30
Codfish cakes, fried	2 small	0
Crab, deviled (2″ diameter)	1 cup	113
Imperial	1 cup	132
Fish sticks	4	12
Lobster Newburg	1 cup	218
Salad	½ cup	94
Oyster stew, made with milk	1 cup	280
Tuna salad	1 cup	41
Fruit		
Apple juice, fresh or canned	1 cup	15
Apples, raw	1 large	10
Canned or stewed	1 cup	10
Apricots, canned in syrup	1 cup	30
Dried, uncooked	1 cup	90
Fresh	3 medium	20
Nectar, or juice	1 cup	20

Calcium Content in Milligram of Selected Foods

Food	Portion	Calcium Content
Avocado	½ large	10
Banana	1 medium	10
Blackberries, fresh	1 cup	45
Blueberries, canned	1 cup	20
Fresh	1 cup	20
Frozen	1 cup	20
Cantaloupe	½ medium	40
Cherries, canned, pitted, Unsweetened	1 cup	40
Fresh, raw	1 cup	35
Dates, dried	1 cup	105
Figs		
Fresh, raw	3 medium	55
Stewed or canned with syrup	3 medium	10
Fruit cocktail, canned	1 cup	20
Grapefruit, canned sections	1 cup	30
Fresh, (5″ diameter)	½	15
Juice	1 cup	20
Grapes, concord	1 cup	15
Muscat	1 cup	20
Grape juice, bottled	1 cup	30
Lemon juice	½ cup	10
Lemonade, frozen (concentrate)	6 oz.	10
Limeade, frozen (concentrate)	6 oz.	20
Olives, canned, large, green	10	25
Canned, large, ripe	10	60
Oranges, fresh, large	1	55–80
Orange juice, with added calcium	6 oz.	200–300
Papaya, fresh, cubed	1 cup	30
Peaches, canned, sliced	1 cup	10
Fresh	1 medium	14
Pears, canned, sweetened	1 cup	15
Raw, 2½″ × 3″	1 medium	20
Persimmons, Japanese	1 medium	10
Pineapple, canned, sliced	1 cup	30
Crushed	1 cup	30
Raw, diced	1 cup	25
Plums, canned in syrup	1 cup	25
Raw, 2″ diameter	1	10
Prunes, cooked (unsweetened)	1 cup	50
Prune juice (unsweetened)	1 cup	35

Calcium Content in Milligram of Selected Foods

Food	Portion	Calcium Content
Raisins, dried	½ cup	50
Raspberries, frozen	½ cup	15
Rhubarb, cooked (sweetened)	1 cup	120
Strawberries, frozen	1 cup	35
Raw	1 cup	35
Tangerines, fresh	1 medium	35
Watermelon, 4″ × 8″	1 wedge	30
Meat and Poultry		
Bacon, cooked crisp and drained	2	2
Beef, corned beef	3 oz.	20
Chuck, pot roast	3 oz.	9
Dried, chipped beef	3 oz.	15
Ground lean	3 oz.	11
Hamburger, commercial	3 oz.	10
Roast beef (oven-cooked)	3 oz.	10
Steak, round	3 oz.	13
Steak, sirloin	3 oz.	10
Chicken, broiled	3 oz.	7
Fried, breast, leg or thigh	3 oz.	7
Roasted	3 oz.	7
Duck	3 oz.	9
Lamb, chop, broiled	4 oz.	11
Pork, chop, thick	3 oz.	8
Ham, canned	2 oz.	5
Turkey, roasted	3 oz.	9
Veal, cutlet, broiled	3 oz.	9
Beef, cooked	1 slice	12
Beef and cheese enchiladas	8 oz.	310
Chili con carne with beans	1 cup	82
Chili con carne without beans	1 cup	14
Pot pie (4½″ diameter)	1 pie	35
Ravioli, with beef	7½ oz.	34
Spaghetti, meatballs, cheese	1 cup	125
Stew, vegetables	1 cup	30
Brains, beef, calf, pork, sheep	3½ oz.	10
Chicken, a la king	1 cup	127
Chow mein	1 cup	58
Devine, prepared with milk	7 oz.	174
Fricassee, prepared	1 cup	14

Calcium Content in Milligram of Selected Foods

Food	Portion	Calcium Content
Chicken (*cont.*)		
Pot pie (4 ½" diameter)	1 pie	40
Frankfurter, beef, 7" long	2	12
Heart, beef, sauteed with oil	3 oz.	6
Calf, 1 large slice	3 oz.	3
Chicken	3 medium	3
Lamb, 2 slices	3 oz.	12
Pork, 2 slices	3 oz.	3
Liverwurst	2 oz.	4
Luncheon meats, Bologna, (4" diameter)	2 slices	7
Dried chipped beef	3 oz.	15
Ham	2 oz.	5
Roast beef	1 slice	12
Pork, ham, canned, spiced	2 oz.	5
Ham, croquette	1	45
Ham, luncheon meat	2 oz.	5
Pork, bacon, cooked and drained	2	2
Sausage, bulk	3 ½ oz.	7
Sweetbreads, calf, braised	3 ½ oz.	7
Tongue, beef	3 oz.	7
Nuts		
Almonds, dried	½ cup	170
Roasted and salted	½ cup	185
Brazil nuts	½ cup	130
Cashews	½ cup	30
Coconut, shredded	½ cup	10
Peanut butter (commercial)	⅓ cup	50
Peanuts, roasted	⅓ cup	40
Pecans, raw	½ cup	35
Sesame seeds, dry	½ cup	85
Sunflower seeds	½ cup	90
Walnuts, raw	½ cup	60
Oils, Fats, and Shortening		
Butter	1 Tbsp.	35
Hydrogenated cooking fat	1 cup	0
Lard	1 cup	0
Margarine	1 Tbsp.	5
Margarine	½ cup	20

Calcium Content in Milligram of Selected Foods

Food	Portion	Calcium Content
Mayonnaise	1 Tbsp.	5
Oils		
Corn, safflower, soy bean oils	1 Tbsp.	0
Olive oil	1 Tbsp.	0
Peanut oil	1 Tbsp.	0
Salad dressing		
Blue and Roquefort cheese	2 Tbsp.	25
French	2 Tbsp.	5
Italian	2 Tbsp.	5
Russian	2 Tbsp.	5
Thousand Island	2 Tbsp.	5
Soups, Canned and Prepared		
Asparagus (prepared with milk)	8 oz.	175
Bean with pork, (prepared with milk)	8 oz.	285
Beef noodle	8 oz.	15
Beef vegetable	8 oz.	15
Broccoli, (prepared with milk)	8 oz.	285
Cheese, (prepared with milk)	8 oz.	275
Chicken or Turkey, (without milk)	8 oz.	25
Chicken gumbo	8 oz.	40
Chicken noodle	8 oz.	10
Chicken with rice	8 oz.	5
Chicken vegetable	8 oz.	15
Clam chowder, Manhattan type	8 oz.	75
Clam chowder, New England type	8 oz.	190
Cream soups, chicken, turkey, celery, mushroom, potato	8 oz.	100–215
Minestrone	8 oz.	35
Split-pea, with milk	8 oz.	180
Split-pea, with water	8 oz.	30
Tomato, with milk	8 oz.	170
Tomato, with water	8 oz.	15
Vegetable beef	8 oz.	10
Vegetable, vegetarian	8 oz.	20
Vegetables		
Artichoke, globe	1 large	60
Asparagus, green	6 spears	20

Calcium Content in Milligram of Selected Foods

Food	Portion	Calcium Content
Beans, baked beans	1 cup	150
Black beans	1 cup	270
Garbanzo beans, canned	1 cup	150
Green beans, snap	1 cup	80
Lima, cooked	1 cup	80
Navy, baked with port	1 cup	95
Red kidney beans, canned	1 cup	75
Bean sprouts, uncooked	1 cup	20
Beets, cooked	1 cup	25
Beets, greens, steamed	1 cup	145
Broccoli, steamed	1 cup	135
Brussels sprouts, steamed	1 cup	50
Cabbage, as coleslaw (with Mayonnaise)	1 cup	50
Sauerkraut, canned	1 cup	85
Steamed cabbage	1 cup	65
Carrots, cooked, diced	1 cup	50
Raw, grated	1 cup	40
Strips, from raw	2 oz.	20
Cauliflower, steamed	1 cup	25
Celery, cooked, diced	1 cup	50
Stalk, raw	1 cup	45
Chard, steamed, leaves	1 cup	130
Collards, steamed	1 cup	35
Corn, steamed	1 ear	5
Canned	1 cup	10
Fritters	1	22
Cucumbers, 1/8″ slices	1 cup	5
Dandelion greens, steamed	1 cup	300
Eggplant, steamed	1 cup	25
Endive	1 cup	45
Kale, steamed	1 cup	205
Lentils	1 cup	50
Lettuce, green, iceberg	1/4 head	20
Mushrooms, raw	1 cup	10
Mustard greens, steamed	1 cup	200
Okra, steamed	1 cup	150
Onions, cooked	1 cup	50
Raw, green	1 cup	65
Parsnips, steamed	1 cup	70

Calcium Content in Milligram of Selected Foods

Food	Portion	Calcium Content
Peas, green, canned	1 cup	50
Fresh, steamed	1 cup	35
Frozen	1 cup	30
Pickles, cucumber, dill, large	1 pickle	35
Potatoes, baked	1 medium	15
Chips	10	10
French fries	10	10
Mashed with milk and butter	1 cup	70
Potato salad	1 cup	80
Scalloped with cheese	1 cup	310
Steamed	1 medium	15
Sweet potato, baked with skin	1 potato	40
Sweet potato, canned	1 can	85
Rutabagas	½ cup	50
Soybeans	1 cup	130
Curd, (2½″ × 2¾″)	1 piece	155
Spinach, steamed	1 cup	170
Squash, summer	1 cup	45
Tomatoes, canned, whole	1 cup	55
Catsup	1 Tbsp.	5
Juice	1 cup	20
Raw	1 large	25
Turnip greens, steamed	1 cup	270
Watercress, raw, chopped finely	1 cup	190
McDonalds		
Egg McMuffin	1	226
Hotcakes with butter	1 serving	103
Scrambled eggs	1 serving	61
Pork sausage	1 serving	16
English muffin with butter	1	117
Hashbrown potatoes	1 serving	5.33
Biscuit with spread	1	74
Biscuit with sausage	1	82
Biscuit with sausage and egg	1	119
Sausage McMuffin	1	196
Apple Danish	1	14
Iced Cheese Danish	1	32.9
Cinnamon Raisin Danish	1	35
Raspberry Danish	1	14.2

Calcium Content in Milligram of Selected Foods

Food	Portion	Calcium Content
Hamburger	1 (100 g)	84
Cheeseburger	1 (114 g)	169
Quarter pounder	1 (160 g)	98
Quarter pounder with cheese	1 (186 g)	255
Big Mac	1 (200 g)	203
Filet-O-Fish	1 (143 g)	133
McD. L. T.	1 (254 g)	250
Chicken McNuggets	109 g	11
French fries	1 serving	9
Apple pie	1 (85 g)	14
Vanilla milkshake	1 (291 g)	329
Chocolate milkshake	1 (291 g)	320
Strawberry milkshake	1 (290 g)	322
Soft serve ice cream and cone	1 (115 g)	183
Strawberry sundae	1 (164 g)	174
Hot fudge sundae	1 (165 g)	215
Hot caramel sundae	1 (165 g)	200
McDonaldland cookies	67 g	12
Chocolaty Chip cookies	69 g	29
Burger King		
Burger King Whopper Sandwich	1	84
Whopper with Cheese	1	215
Double Beef Whopper	1	95
Double Beef Whopper with Cheese	1	226
Whopper Jr. Sandwich	1	40
Whopper Jr. with Cheese	1	105
Bacon Double Cheeseburger	1	168
Hamburger	1	37
Cheeseburger	1	102
Whaler Sandwich	1	46
Ham and Cheese Sandwich	1	195
Chicken Sandwich	1	79
Salad, plain	1 serving	18
With House Dressing	1 serving	37
With Blue Cheese	1 serving	44
With Thousand Island	1 serving	66
With Reduced Calorie Italian	1 serving	42
Breakfast Croissan'wich	1	40
Bacon Egg, Cheese	1	136

Calcium Content in Milligram of Selected Foods

Food	Portion	Calcium Content
Breakfast Croissan'wich (*cont.*)		
Sausage, Egg, Cheese	1	145
Ham, Egg, Cheese	1	136
Scrambled Egg Platter	1 serving	101
With sausage	1 serving	112
With bacon	1 serving	103
French Toast Sticks	1 serving	77
Great Danish	1	91
Onion Rings, regular	1 serving	124
Milk		
2% lowfat	1 cup	297
Whole	1 cup	290
Shakes, medium		
Vanilla	1	295
Chocolate	1	260
Vanilla (syrup added)	1	NA
Chocolate (syrup added)	1	248
Sandwiches		
Bacon, lettuce and tomato on white bread	1	53
Chicken salad on white bread	1	50
Corned beef on rye bread	1	50
Cream cheese and jelly on white bread	1	60
Egg salad on white bread	1	65
Ham on white bread	1	40
Hot dog on bun	1	65
Peanut butter and jelly on white bread	1	70
Roast beef on white bread	1	60
Tuna salad on white bread	1	48
Combination Foods		
Beans and franks	8 oz.	122
Beef pie	8 oz.	32
Beef vegetable stew	8 oz.	29
Beef stroganoff	6 oz.	24
Cabbage rolls	8 oz.	55
Cannelloni, beef, tomato sauce	8 ¼ oz.	298
Chicken, cheese sauce	8 ¼ oz.	389
Shrimp, cheese sauce	8 ¼ oz.	490

Calcium Content in Milligram of Selected Foods

Food	Portion	Calcium Content
Chicken a la king	8 oz.	127
Chicken and noodles	8 oz.	26
Chicken and rice	8 oz.	122
Chicken parmigiana	7 oz.	174
Chicken pie	8 oz.	70
Chili con carne with beans	8 oz.	90
Without beans	8 oz.	80
Chicken chow mein	8 oz.	40–50
Enchiladas, beef and cheese	8 oz.	309
Enchiladas, cheese	12 oz.	425
Corn fritter	3½ oz.	64
Corned beef hash	10 oz.	65
Macaroni and cheese	12 oz.	220
Lasagna and cheese	8 oz.	220
Miscellaneous		
Featherweight baking powder	1 Tbsp.	1500

Calcium Supplements

Since not all calcium supplements are alike, care must be taken in selecting one at the drugstrore. The type of calcium salt in the formulation (as well as any other active ingredients) determines the amount that is absorbed by your body. For example, you may need to take 3 grams (3,000 mg) of calcium carbonate to obtain the 1,500 mg necessary to fulfill the needs of a postmenopausal woman.

The major types of calcium salts available include: calcium carbonate (oyster shell calcium), calcium gluconate, calcium citrate, and calcium lactate. They are present in varying dosages; with or without vitamin D, phosphorous, and other vitamins or minerals.

The best approach to selecting one is to read the label to determine how much *elemental calcium* is present. (A calcium tablet may contain 1,250 mg of calcium carbonate but that's only equivalent to 500 mg of usable calcium.) Next, check the label to find out what percentage of the RDA (Recommended Daily Allowance) for calcium the tablet provides. Five hundred mg of elemental calcium in calcium carbonate provides 50 percent of the RDA for menstruating women. (Pregnant women and postmenopausal women need more.) Don't attempt to fulfill all of your calcium RDA via a pill, because combining it with dietary calcium may cause you to take in too much. This is not only a waste of money, but it can be dangerous.

Preparations vary in terms of their side effects. The most common serious side effect from excess calcium intake is the formation of kidney stones. This may be minimized by trying to obtain most of your calcium needs through good nutrition rather than supplements, and by drinking eight ounces of water with your tablet.

Finally, certain drugs, including: anticonvulsants, diuretics, corticosteroids, calcium channel blocker-type heart medications, digitalis, and antibiotics (such as tetracycline), interact with calcium. *Calcium supplements should not be taken with these medications.* Make sure to check with your doctor before starting calcium supplements.

Vitamin D

The RDA for vitamin D is 400 I.U. (international units). Our bodies synthesize the vitamin D we need by daily exposure to sunlight. Other sources of vitamin D include: fish liver oil, eggs, and vitamin D–fortified milk. Supplements are generally not necessary, and may lead to harmful overdoses.

The First Step in Eating Right Is Buying Right: A Guide to Choosing Low-Fat, Low-Cholesterol Foods

Variety is the spice of life. Choose foods every day from each of the following food groups. Choose different foods from within groups, especially foods low in saturated fat and cholesterol (the **Choose** column). As a guide, the recommended daily number of servings for adults is listed for each food group. But you'll have to decide on the number of servings you need to lose or maintain your weight. If you need help, ask a dietitian or your doctor.

	Choose	Go Easy On	Decrease
Meat, Poultry, Fish, and Shellfish (up to 6 ounces a day)	*Lean cuts* of meat with fat trimmed, like: • beef—round, sirloin, chuck, loin • lamb—leg, arm, loin, rib • pork—tenderloin, leg (fresh), shoulder (arm or picnic) • veal—all trimmed cuts except ground • poultry without skin • fish, shellfish		"Prime" grade *Fatty cuts* of meat like: • beef—corned beef brisket, regular ground, short ribs • pork—spareribs, blade roll Goose, domestic duck Organ meats, like liver, kidney, sweetbreads, brain Sausage, bacon Regular luncheon meats Frankfurters Caviar, roe
Dairy Products (2 servings a day; 3 servings for women who are pregnant or breast feeding)	Skim milk, 1% milk, low-fat buttermilk, low-fat evaporated or nonfat milk Low-fat yogurt and low-fat frozen yogurt Low-fat soft cheeses, like cottage, farmer, pot Cheeses labeled no more than 2 to 6 grams of fat an ounce	2% milk Whole milk Yogurt Part-skim ricotta Part-skim or imitation hard cheeses, like part-skim mozzarella "Light" cream cheese "Light" sour cream	Whole milk like regular, evaporated, condensed Cream, half-and-half, most nondairy creamers and products, real or nondairy whipped cream Cream cheese Ice cream Sour cream Custard-style yogurt Whole-milk ricotta High-fat cheeses, like Neufchatel, Brie, Swiss, American, mozzarella, feta, cheddar, Muenster
Eggs (no more than 3 egg yolks a week)	Egg whites Cholesterol-free egg substitutes		Egg yolks
Fats and Oils (up to 6 to 8 teaspoons a day)	Unsaturated vegetable oils: corn, olive, peanut, rapeseed (canola oil), safflower, sesame, soybean Margarine or shortening made with unsaturated fats listed above: liquid, tub, stick, diet Mayonnaise, salad dressings made with unsaturated fats listed above Low-fat dressings	Nuts and seeds Avocados and olives	Butter, coconut oil, palm kernel oil, palm oil, lard, bacon fat Margarine or shortening made with saturated fats listed above Dressings made with egg yolk

	Choose	Go Easy On	Decrease
Breads, Cereals, Pasta, Rice, Dried Peas and Beans (6 to 11 servings a day) 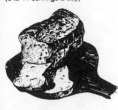	Breads, like white, whole wheat, pumpernickel, and rye breads; pita; bagels; English muffins; sandwich buns; dinner rolls; rice cakes Low-fat crackers, like matzo, bread sticks, rye krisp, saltines, zwieback Hot cereals, most cold dry cereals Pasta, like plain noodles, spaghetti, macaroni Any grain rice Dried peas and beans, like split peas, black-eyed peas, chick peas, kidney beans, navy beans, lentils, soybeans, soybean curd (tofu)	Store-bought pancakes, waffles, biscuits, muffins, cornbread	Croissants, butter rolls, sweet rolls, Danish pastry, doughnuts Most snack crackers, like cheese crackers, butter crackers, those made with saturated fats Granola-type cereals made with saturated fats Pasta and rice prepared with cream, butter, or cheese sauces; egg noodles
Fruits and Vegetables (2 to 4 servings of fruit and 3 to 5 servings of vegetables a day)	Fresh, frozen, canned, or dried fruits and vegetables		Vegetables prepared in butter, cream, or sauce
Sweets and Snacks (avoid too many sweets) 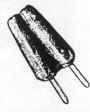	Low-fat frozen desserts, like sherbet, sorbet, Italian ice, frozen yogurt, popsicles Low-fat cakes, like angel food cake Low-fat cookies, like fig bars, gingersnaps Low-fat candy, like jelly beans, hard candy Low-fat snacks, like plain popcorn, pretzels Nonfat beverages, like carbonated drinks, juices, tea, coffee	Frozen desserts, like ice milk Homemade cakes, cookies, and pies using unsaturated oils sparingly Fruit crisps and cobblers Potato and corn chips prepared with unsaturated vegetable oil	High-fat frozen desserts, like ice cream, frozen tofu High-fat cakes, like most store-bought, pound, and frosted cakes Store-bought pies Most store-bought cookies Most candy, like chocolate bars Potato and corn chips prepared with saturated fat Buttered popcorn High-fat beverages, like frappes, milkshakes, floats, and eggnogs

Label Ingredients

To avoid too much fat, saturated fat, or cholesterol, go easy on products that list first any fat, oil, or ingredients higher in saturated fat or cholesterol. Choose more often those products that contain ingredients lower in saturated fat or cholesterol.

Prepared by the National Heart, Lung, and Blood Institute.

Ingredients Lower in Saturated Fat or Cholesterol
Carob, cocoa
Oils, like corn, cottonseed, olive, safflower, sesame, soybean, or sunflower
Nonfat dry milk, nonfat dry milk solids, skim milk

Ingredients Higher in Saturated Fat or Cholesterol
Chocolate
Animal fat, like bacon, beef, ham, lamb, meat, pork, chicken or turkey fats, butter, lard
Coconut, coconut oil, palm kernel or palm oil
Cream
Egg and egg-yolk solids
Hardened fat or oil
Hydrogenated vegetable oil
Shortening or vegetable shortening
Unspecified vegetable oil (could be coconut, palm kernel, palm)

Bibliography

Preface

1. Budoff, Penny, *No More Menstrual Cramps and Other Good News* (New York: Putnam, 1980), pp. 178–9.

2. Cutler, Winnifred B., *Hysterectomy: Before and After* (New York: Harper & Row, 1988), p. 2.

3. Giustini, F.G. and Keefer, F. J., *Understanding Hysterectomy: A Woman's Guide* (New York: Walker and Company, 1979), p. 44.

4. Irwin, Kathleen L., et al., "Hysterectomy among Women of Reproductive Age, United States, Update for 1981–1982," *Morbidity and Mortality Weekly Report Center for Disease Surveillance Summary for 1986*, 35:1, pp. 1SS–6SS.

5. Lyons, Albert S. and Petrucelli, R. Joseph, *Medicine: An Illustrated History* (New York: Abradale, 1987), p. 217.

6. Pokras, Robert and Hufnagel, Vicki G., "Hysterectomies in the United States: 1965–1984," *Vital and Health Statistics*, U.S. Department of Health and Human Services, National Health Survey, 13:92, pp. 1–32.

7. Sandberg, Sonja I., et al., "Elective Hysterectomy: Benefits, Risks, and Costs," *Medical Care* (September 1985), 23:9, p. 1068.

8. Scully, Diane, *Men Who Control Women's Health: The Miseducation of Obstetrician-Gynecologists* (Boston: Houghton Mifflin, 1980), p. 141.

9. Stokes, Naomi Miller, *The Castrated Woman: What your Doctor Won't Tell You About Hysterectomy* (New York: Franklin Watts, 1986), p.49.

Chapter One

1. Budoff, Penny, *No More Menstrual Cramps and Other Good News* (New York: Putnam, 1980), pp. 178–9.

2. Bunker, John P., "Elective Hysterectomy: Pro and Con," *The New England Journal of Medicine* (July 29, 1976), 295:5, p. 265.

3. Bunker, John P., "Surgical Manpower: A Comparison of Operations and Surgeons in the United States and in England and Wales," *New England Journal of Medicine* (January 15, 1979), 282:3, pp. 135–44.

4. Cole, Philip and Berlin, Joyce, "Elective Hysterectomy," *American Journal of Obstetrics and Gynecology* (September 15, 1977), 129:2, pp. 117–29.

5. "Cost and Quality of Health Care: Unnecessary Surgery," Report by the Subcommittee on Oversight and Investigations of the Committee on Interstate and Foreign Commerce (Washington, DC: U.S. Government Printing Office, 1976).

6. Dicker, Richard C., et al., "Hysterectomy Among Women of Reproductive Age: Trends in the United States,1970–1978," *Journal of the American Medical Association* (July 16, 1982), 248:3, pp. 323–7.

7. Domenighetti, Gianfranco and Luraschi, Pierangelo, "Hysterectomy and the Sex of the Gynecologist," Letter to the Editor *New England Journal of Medicine* (December 5, 1985), 313:23, p. 1482.

8. Dyck, Frank J., et al., "Effect of Surveillance on the Number of Hysterectomies in the Province of Saskatchewan," *New England Journal of Medicine* (June 9, 1977), 296:23, pp. 1326–28.

9. Evans, W. A., *Dr. Evans' How to Keep Well Book: A Health Book for the Home* (New York: D. Appleton and Company, 1917), pp. 965–6.

10. Giustini, F. G., and Keefer, F. J., *Understanding Hysterectomy: A Woman's Guide* (New York: Walker and Company, 1979), pp. 13–14, 39, 47.

11. Harrison, Michelle, *A Woman in Residence* (New York: Random House, 1982), p. 32.

12. Lyons, Albert S. and Petrucelli, R. Joseph, *Medicine: An Illustrated History* (New York: Abradale, 1987), p. 529.

13. Notman, Malkah T. and Nadelson, Carol C., *The Woman Patient: Medical and Psychological Interfaces* (New York: Plenum, 1978), p. 222.

14. Novak, Edmund R., Jones, Georgeanna S., and Jones, Howard, *Novak's Textbook of Gynecology* (Baltimore: Williams and Wilkins, 1975), p. 113.

15. Pernick, Martin S., *A Calculus of Suffering: Pain, Professionalism and Anesthesia in Nineteenth Century America* (New York: Columbia University Press, 1985).

16. Pokras, Robert and Hufnagel, Vicki G., "Hysterectomies in the United States: 1965–1984," *Vital and Health Statistics*, U.S. Department of Health and Human Services, National Health Survey, 13:92, p. 3.

17. Roeske, Nancy C., "Hysterectomy and the Quality of a Woman's Life," Editorial, *Archives of Internal Medicine* (February 1979), 139:2, pp. 146–7.

18. Rutkow, Ira M. and Zuidema, George D., "Unnecessary Surgery: An Update," *Surgery* (November 1978), 84:5, p. 672.

19. Sandberg, Sonja I., et al., "Elective Hysterectomy: Benefits, Risks, and Costs," *Medical Care* (September 1985), 23:9, p. 1067.

20. Scott, Russell C., *The World of the Gynecologist*, in Scully, Diane, *Men Who Control Women's Health: The Miseducation of Obstetrician-Gynecologists* (Boston: Houghton Mifflin, 1980), p. 102.

21. Scully, Diane, *Men Who Control Women's Health: The Miseducation of Obstetrician-Gynecologists* (Boston: Houghton Mifflin, 1980), pp. 25–60, 103–4, 141–5.

22. Stage, Sarah, *Female Complaints: Lydia Pinkham and the Business of Women's Medicine* (New York: Norton, 1979), pp. 77–8.

23. Stokes, Naomi Miller, *The Castrated Woman: What Your Doctor Won't Tell You About Hysterectomy* (New York: Franklin Watts, 1986), pp. 143–50.

24. Stumpf, Paul G., "Prophylactic Hysterectomy at Oophorectomy in Young Women," Letter to the Editor, *Journal of the American Medical Association* (September 7, 1984), 252:9, p. 1129.

25. Wennberg, John and Gittelsohn, Alan, "Variations in Medical Care among Small Areas," *Scientific American* (April 1982), 246:4, pp. 120–34.

26. Wright, Ralph C., "Hysterectomy: Past, Present and Future," *Obstetrics and Gynecology* (April 1969), 3:33, pp. 560–3.

Chapter Two

1. Boston Women's Health Collective, *The New Our Bodies, Ourselves* (New York: Simon & Schuster, 1984), pp. 203–19, 443–7.

2. Clarke, Edward H., *Sex in Education, or A Fair Chance for Girls* (Boston: Robert Brothers, 1873), p. 33, as cited in Stage, Sarah, *Female Complaints: Lydia Pinkham and the Business of Women's Medicine* (New York: Norton, 1979), p. 69.

3. Crouch, James E., *Functional Human Anatomy*, 3rd ed. (Philadelphia: Lea and Febiger, 1978), pp. 561–609.

4. Cutler, Winnefred B., *Hysterectomy: Before and After* (New York: Harper & Row, 1988), pp.14, 34, 41.

5. Ezrin, Calvin, Godden, John O., and Volpé, Robert, *Systematic Endocrinology,* 2nd ed. (New York, Harper & Row, 1979), pp. 258–331.

6. Guyton, Arthur C., *Textbook of Medical Physiology* (Philadelphia: Saunders, 1976), pp. 1086–103.

7. Madaras, Lynda and Patterson, Jane, with Schick, Peter, *Womancare: A Gynecological Guide to Your Body* (New York: Avon, 1984), pp. 50–76.

8. Silverstein, Alvin, *Human Anatomy and Physiology,* 2nd ed. (New York: Wiley, 1983), pp. 623–35.

9. Todd, W. Duane and Tapley, Donald F., eds., *The Columbia University College of Physicians and Surgeons Complete Guide to Pregnancy* (New York: Crown, 1988), p. 213.

Chapter Three

1. Andreotti, Rochelle F., et al., "Ultrasound and Magnetic Resonance Imaging of Pelvic Masses," *Surgery, Gynecology and Obstetrics* (April 1988), 166:4, pp. 327–32.

2. Baird, David and West, Christine, "Medical Management of Fibroids," *British Medical Journal* (June 18, 1988), 296:6638, pp. 1684–5.

3. Baltarowich, Oksana H., et al., "Pitfalls in the Sonographic Diagnosis of Fibroids," *American Journal of Radiology* (October 1988), 151, pp. 725–8.

4. Ben-Baruch, G., Schiff, E. Menashe, Y., and Menczer, J., "Immediate and Late Outcome of Vaginal Myomectomy for Prolapsed Pedunculated Submucous Myoma," *Obstetrics and Gynecology* (December 1988), 72:6, pp. 858–60.

5. Boston Women's Health Book Collective, *The New Our Bodies, Ourselves* (New York: Simon & Schuster, 1984), p. 510.

6. Brooks, Philip G., et al., "Resectoscopy: Mastering the Challenges," *Contemporary OB/GYN* (August 1989), pp. 131–48.

7. Cooke, Cynthia W. and Dworkin, Susan, *The Ms. Guide to a Woman's Health* (New York: Berkley, 1979), pp. 364–5.

8. Corfman, Randle S., "Indications for Hysteroscopy," *Obstetrics and Gynecology Clinics of North America* (March 1988), 15:1, pp. 41–9.

9. Coutinho, Elsimar, Boulanger, Genevieve, Azadian, and Gonçalves, Maria Tereza, "Regression of Uterine Leiomyomas After Treatment with Gestrinone, An Antiestrogen, Antiprogesterone," *American Journal of Obstetrics and Gynecology* (October 1986), 155:4, pp. 761–7.

10. Danforth, David N. and Scott, James, R., *Obstetrics/Gynecology* (Philadelphia: Lippincott, 1986), pp. 1079–80.

11. Droegemueller, William, et al., *Comprehensive Gynecology* (Washington, DC: Mosby, 1987), pp. 459–65.

12. Dudiak, C. M., et al., "Uterine Leiomyomas in the Infertile Patient: Preoperative Localization with MR Imaging versus US and Hysterosalpingography," *Radiology* (June 1988), 167:3, pp.627–30.

13. Goldfarb, Herbert A., "D&C Results Improved by Hysteroscopy," *New Jersey Medicine* (April 1989), 86:4, pp. 277–9.

14. Goldrath, Milton H., "Vaginal Removal of the Pedunculated Submucous Myoma: The Use of Laminaria," *Obstetrics and Gynecology* (October 1987), 70:10, pp. 670–1.

15. Goldrath, M. and Sherman, A. I., "Office Hysteroscopy and Suction Curettage: Can We Eliminate the Hospital Diagnostic Dilation and Curettage?" *American Journal of Obstetrics and Gynecology* (1985), 152, pp. 220–9.

16. Harrison, Michelle, *A Woman In Residence* (New York: Random House, 1982), pp. 35, 59, 216.

17. Healy, David L., et al., "Toward Removing Uterine Fibroids without Surgery: Subcutaneous Infusion of a Luteinizing Hormone–Releasing Hormone Agonist Commencing in the Luteal Phase," *Journal of Clinical Endocrinology and Metabolism* (1986), 63:1, pp. 619–24.

18. Hricak, Hedvig, "MRI of the Female Pelvis: A Review," *American Journal of Radiology* (June 1986), 146, pp. 1115–22.

19. Hricak, Hedvig, et al., "Uterine Leiomyomas: Correlation of MR, Histopathologic Findings, and Symptoms," *Radiology* (February 1986), 158:2, pp. 385–91.

20. Kistner, Robert, *Gynecology: Principles and Practices* (Chicago: Year Book Medical Publishers), pp. 196–209.

21. "Uterine Fibroids: Medical Treatment or Surgery?" Editorial, *The Lancet* (November 22, 1986), 2: 8517, p. 1197.

22. Lavy, Gad, "Hysteroscopy as a Diagnostic Aid," *Obstetrics and Gynecology Clinics of North America* (March 1988), 15:1, pp. 61–72.

23. LiPuma, Joseph P., et al., "Magnetic Resonance Imaging of the Genitourinary Tract," *Urologic Clinics of North America* (August 1986), 13:3, pp. 531–50.

24. Loffer, Franklin D., "Hysteroscopy with Selective Endometrial Sampling Compared with D&C for Abnormal Uterine Bleeding: The Value of a Negative View," *Obstetrics and Gynecology* (January 1989), 73:1, pp. 16–9.

25. Loffer, Franklin D., "Laser Ablation of the Endometrium," *Obstetrics and Gynecology Clinics of North America* (March 1988), 15:1, pp. 77–89.

26. McLachlan, Robert I., Healy, David L., and Burger, Henry G., "Clinical Aspects of LHRH Analogues in Gynaecology: A Review," *British Journal of Obstetrics and Gynaecology* (May 1986), 93:5, pp. 431–54.

27. Madaras, Lynda and Patterson, Jane, with Schick, Peter, *Womancare: A Gynecological Guide to Your Body* (New York: Avon, 1981).

28. Makarainen, Leo and Olavi, Ylikorkala, "Primary and Myoma-Induced Menorrhagia: Role of Prostaglandins and Effects of Ibuprofen," *British Journal of Obstetrics and Gynaecology* (September 1986), 93:9, pp. 974–8.

29. Mark, Alexander S., et al., "Adenomyosis and Leiomyoma: Differential Diagnosis with MR Imaging," *Radiology* (May 1987), 163:2, pp. 527–9.

30. Mendelson, Ellen B., et al., "Gynecologic Imaging: Comparison of Transabdominal and Transvaginal Sonography," *Radiology* (February 1988), 166:2, pp. 321–4.

31. Napoli, Maryann, "Medical Breakthrough: Laser Hysterectomy," *Ms.* (March 1986), pp. 30–1.

32. Neuwirth, Robert S., "Hysteroscopic Management of Symptomatic Submucous Fibroids," *Obstetrics and Gynecology* (October 1983), 62:4, pp. 509–11.

33. Parazzini, Fabio, et al., "Epidemiologic Characteristics of Women with Uterine Fibroids: A Case-Control Study," *Obstetrics and Gynecology* (December 1988), 72:6, pp. 853–7.

34. Ross, Ron K., et al., "Risk Factors for Uterine Fibroids: Reduced Risk Associated with Oral Contraceptives," *British Medical Journal* (August 9, 1986), 293:6543, pp. 359–62.

35. Russell, Jeffrey B., "History and Development of Hysteroscopy," *Obstetrics and Gynecology Clinics of North America* (March 1988), 15:1, pp. 1–11.

36. Shapiro, Bruce S., "Instrumentation in Hysteroscopy," *Obstetrics and Gynecology Clinics of North America* (March 1988), 15:1, pp. 13–21.

37. Stage, Sarah, *Female Complaints: Lydia Pinkham and the Business of Women's Medicine* (New York: Norton, 1979), pp. 70–1.

38. Valle, Rafael F., "Future Growth and Development of Hysteroscopy," *Obstetrics and Gynecology Clinics of North America* (March 1988), 15:1, pp. 113–26.

39. vanLeusden, H.A.I.M., "Rapid Reduction of Uterine Myomas After Short-term Treatment with Microencapsulated D-Trp-LHRH," *The Lancet* (November 22, 1986), 2:8517, p. 1213.

40. Wheeler, James M. and DeCherney, Alan H., "Office Hysteroscopy," *Obstetrics and Gynecology Clinics of North America* (March 1988), 15:1, pp. 29–39.

41. Willson, J. Robert and Carrington, Elsie Reid, *Obstetrics and Gynecology* (Washington, DC: Mosby, 1987), pp. 649–55.

42. Ylikorkala, O. and Pekonen, Fredrika, "Naproxen Reduces Idiopathic But Not Fibromyoma-Induced Menorrhagia," *Obstetrics and Gynecology* (July 1986), 68:1, pp. 10–12.

Chapter Four

1. Barbieri, Robert L., "New Therapy for Endometriosis," *The New England Journal of Medicine* (February 25, 1988), 318:8, pp. 512–13.

2. Bohlman, Mark E., Ensor, Robert E., and Sanders, Roger C., "Sonographic Findings in Adenomyosis of the Uterus," *American Journal of Radiology* (April 1987), 148, pp. 765–6.

3. Boston Women's Health Book Collective, *The New Our Bodies, Ourselves* (New York: Simon & Schuster, 1984), pp. 480–1, 500–2.

4. Breitkopf, Lyle and Bakoulis, Marion Gordon, *Coping with Endometriosis* (New York: Prentice Hall, 1988).

5. Cramer, Daniel W., et al., "The Relation of Endometriosis to Menstrual Characteristics, Smoking, and Exercise," *Journal of the American Medical Association* (April 11, 1986), 255:14, pp. 1904–8.

6. Davis, Gordon D. and Brooks, Robert A., "Excision of Pelvic Endometriosis with the Carbon Dioxide Laser Laparoscope," *Obstetrics and Gynecology* (November 1988), 72:5, pp. 816–19.

7. Davis, Gordon D., "Management of Endometriosis and Its Associated Adhesions with the CO_2 Laser Laparoscope," *Obstetrics and Gynecology* (September 1986), 68:3, pp. 422–5.

8. Droegemueller, William, *Comprehensive Gynecology* (Washington, DC: Mosby, 1987), pp. 493–514.

9. Fayez, Jamil A., Collazo, Louis M., and Vernon, Cheryl, "Comparison of Different Modalities of Treatment for Minimal and Mild Endometriosis," *American Journal of Obstetrics and Gynecology* (October 1988), 159:4, pp. 927–31.

10. Fedele, Luigi, et al., "Serum CA 125 Measurements in the Diagnosis of Endometriosis Recurrence," *Obstetrics and Gynecology* (July 1988), 72:1, pp. 19–22.

11. Few, Barbara J., "Treating Endometriosis with Nafarelin," *Maternal and Child Nursing* (September/October 1988), 13:5, p. 323.

12. Goldfarb, Herbert A., "The Use of the Carbon Dioxide Laser During Laparoscopic Surgery," *New Jersey Medicine* (January 1988), 85:1, pp. 27–8.

13. Haber, G. M. and Behelak, Y. F., "Preliminary Report on the Use of Tamoxifen in the Treatment of Endometriosis," *American Journal of Obstetrics and Gynecology* (March 1987), 156:3, pp. 582–5.

14. Henze, Milan R., et al., "Administration of Nasal Nafarelin as Compared with Oral Danazol for Endometriosis," *The New England Journal of Medicine* (February 25, 1988), 318:8, pp. 485–9.

15. Kirshon, Brian and Poindexter, Alfred, "Contraception: A Risk Factor for Endometriosis," *Obstetrics and Gynecology* (June 1988), 71:6, pp. 829–31.

16. Kistner, Robert W., *Gynecology: Principles and Practices* (Chicago: Year Book Medical Publishers, 1986), pp. 393–414.

17. "LHRH Analogues in Endometriosis," *The Lancet* (November 1, 1986), 2:8514, pp. 1016–18.

18. Lemay, André, et al., "Efficacy of Intranasal or Subcutaneous Luteinizing Hormone–Releasing Hormone Agonist Inhibition of Ovarian Function in the Treatment of Endometriosis," *Obstetrics and Gynecology* (February 1988), 158, pp. 233–6.

19. Lockhart, W. E. and Karnaky, Karl John, "Treatment of Endometriosis," *American Journal of Obstetrics and Gynecology* (January 1986), 154:1, pp. 215–16.

20. Luciano, Anthony A., Turksoy, R. Nuran, and Carleo, Judith, "Evaluation of Oral Medroxyprogesterone Acetate in the Treatment of Endometriosis," *Obstetrics and Gynecology* (September 1988), 72:3, pp. 323–6.

21. McLachlan, Robert I., Healy, David L., and Burger, Henry G., "Clinical Aspects of LHRH Analogues in Gynaecology: A Review," *British Journal of Obstetrics and Gynaecology* (May 1986), 93:5, pp. 431–54.

22. Mark, Alexander S., et al., "Adenomyosis and Leiomyoma: Differential Diagnosis with MR Imaging," *Radiology* (May 1987), 163:2, pp. 527–9.

23. Mashahashi, T., et al., "Serum CA 125 Levels in Patients with Endometriosis: Changes in CA 125 Levels During Menstruation," *Obstetrics and Gynecology* (September 1988), 72:3, pp. 328–31.

24. Nishimura, K., et al., "Endometrial Cysts of the Ovary: MR Imaging," *Radiology* (February 1987), 162:2, pp. 315–18.

25. Older, Julia, *Endometriosis* (New York: Scribner, 1984).

26. Peterson, Nancy F. and Rhoe, Joelle, "Endometriosis: Obtaining Relief Via 'Near-Contact' Laparoscopy," *AORN Journal* (October 1988), 48:4, pp. 700–7, 710, 712.

27. Pokras, Robert and Hufnagel, Vicki, "Hysterectomies in the United States: 1965–1984," *Vital and Health Statistics*, U.S. Department of Health and Human Services, National Health Survey: 13:92.

28. Rosenfeld, David L. and Jacob, Jessica, "Subsequent Pregnancies in Previously Infertile Women with Endometriosis," *Obstetrics and Gynecology* (December 1988), 72:6, pp. 908–10.

29. Sampson, J. A., "Intestinal Adenomas of Endometrial Type," *Archives of Surgery* (1922), 5, pp. 217–80.

30. Sampson, J. A., "Peritoneal Endometriosis Due to the Menstrual Dissemination of Endometrial Tissue into the Peritoneal Cavity," *American Journal of Obstetrics and Gynecology* (1927), 14, p. 422.

31. Steingold, K. A., et al., "Treatment of Endometriosis with a Long-Acting Gonadotropin-Releasing Hormone Agonist," *Obstetrics and Gynecology* (March 1987), 69:3, pp. 403–10.

32. Togashi, K., et al., "Adenomyosis: Diagnosis with MR Imaging," *Radiology* (January 1988), 166:1, pp. 111–14.

33. Vasilev, Steven A., et al., "Serum CA 125 Levels in Preoperative Evaluation of Pelvic Masses," *Obstetrics and Gynecology* (May 1988), 71:5, pp. 751–5.

34. Weinstein, Kate, *Living with Endometriosis: How to Cope with the Physical and Emotional Challenges* (Massachusetts: Addison-Wesley, 1987).

Chapter Five

1. Budoff, Penny, *No More Menstrual Cramps and Other Good News* (New York: Putnam, 1980), pp. 189–93.

2. Conn, Howard F., ed., *Current Therapy* (Philadelphia: Saunders, 1981), pp. 904–6.

3. Ezrin, Calvin, Godden, John O., and Volpé, Robert, *Systematic Endocrinology* (Maryland: Harper & Row, 1979), pp. 298–303.

4. Jeffcoate, Sir Norman, *Jeffcoate's Principles of Gynaecology* (London: Butterworth, 1987), pp. 512–31.

5. Madaras, Lynda, Patterson, Jane, with Schick, Peter, *Womancare: A Gynecological Guide to Your Body* (New York: Avon, 1984), pp. 635–40.

6. Neeson, Jean and Stockdale, Connie, *The Practitioner's Handbook of Ambulatory Ob/Gyn* (New York: Wiley, 1981), pp. 219–24.

7. Novak, Edmund R., Jones, Georgeanna S., and Jones, Howard, *Novak's Textbook of Gynecology* (Baltimore: Williams and Wilkins, 1981), pp. 777–95.

8. Worley, Richard J., "Dysfunctional Uterine Bleeding: Clarifying Its Definition, Mechanisms, and Management," *Postgraduate Medicine* (February 15, 1986), 79:3, pp. 101–6.

9. Zimmerman, Ralf, "Dysfunctional Uterine Bleeding," *Obstetrics and Gynecology Clinics of North America* (March 1988), 15:1, pp. 107–10.

Chapter Six

1. American Cancer Society, "Cancer Facts and Figures—1990," pp. 10–11.

2. American Cancer Society, *A Cancer Sourcebook for Nurses* (1981), pp. 79–86.

3. Barber, Hugh R. K., *Manual of Gynecologic Oncology* (Philadelphia: Lippencott, 1989).

4. Budoff, Penny, *No More Menstrual Cramps and Other Good News* (New York, Putnam, 1980), pp. 189–93.

5. Evans, Bergen, ed., *Dictionary of Quotations* (New York: Avenel, 1978), p. 325.

6. Hricak, Hedvig, et al., "Endometrial Carcinoma Staging by MR Imaging," *Radiology* (February 1987), 162:2, pp. 297–305.

7. Madaras, Lynda, Patterson, Jane, with Schick, Peter, *Womancare: A Gynecological Guide to Your Body* (New York: Avon, 1981).

8. Petrek, Jeanne, *A Woman's Guide to the Prevention, Detection, and Treatment of Cancer* (New York: MacMillan, 1985), pp. 34-92.

9. Pokras, Robert and Hufnagel, Vicki, "Hysterectomies in the United States: 1965–1984," *Vital and Health Statistics*, U.S. Department of Health and Human Services, National Health Survey, 13, p. 92.

10. Ross, Ronald K., et al., "Avoidable Nondietary Risk Factors for Cancer," *American Family Physician* (August 1988), 38:2, pp. 153–9.

Chapter Seven

1. Boston Women's Health Collective, *The New Our Bodies, Ourselves* (New York: Simon & Schuster, 1984).

2. Madaras, Lynda, Patterson, Jane, with Schick, Peter, *Womancare: A Gynecological Guide to Your Body* (New York: Avon, 1984).

3. Pokras, Robert and Hufnagel, Vicki, "Hysterectomies in the United States: 1965–1984," *Vital and Health Statistics*, U.S. Department of Health and Human Services, National Health Survey, 13, p. 92.

4. Speert, Harold, *Iconographia Gyniatrica: A Pictorial Hystory of Gynecology and Obstetrics* (Philadelphia: Davis, 1973), pp. 463–4.

5. Stage, Sarah, *Female Complaints: Lydia Pinkham and the Business of Women's Medicine* (New York: Norton, 1979).

6. Sturdee, D. W. and Rushton, D. I., "Caesarian and Post-partum Hysterectomy: 1968–1983," *British Journal of Obstetrics and Gynaecology* (March 1986), 93:3, pp. 270–4.

7. Thonet, R. G. N., "Obstetric Hysterectomy: An 11–Year Experience," *British Journal of Obstetrics and Gynaecology* (August 1986), 93:8, pp. 794–8.

8. Jeffcoate, Sir Norman., *Jeffcoate's Principles of Gynaecology* (London: Butterworth, 1987), pp. 260–74.

Chapter Eight

1. American College of Obstetricians and Gynecologists, "Estrogen Replacement Therapy," *ACOG Technical Bulletin* (April 1986), 93, pp. 1–5.

2. American Psychiatric Association, *Diagnostic and Statistical Manual of Mental Disorders*, 3rd ed., rev. (Washington, DC, 1987), pp. 128–9.

3. Barrett-Conner, Elizabeth, "Estrogen Replacement and Coronary Heart Disease," *Cardiovascular Clinics* (1989), pp.159–72.

4. Barzel, Uriel S., "Estrogens in the Prevention and Treatment of Post-menopausal Osteoporosis," *The American Journal of Medicine* (December 1988), 85, pp. 847–9.

5. Brenner, Paul F., "The Menopausal Syndrome," *Obstetrics and Gynecology* (November 1988), 72:5, pp. 6S–11S.

6. Budoff, Penny, *No More Hot Flashes and Other Good News* (New York: Putnam, 1983), pp. 114–15.

7. Castelli, W., "Epidemiology of Coronary Heart Disease: The Framingham Study," *American Journal of Medicine* (1984), 76, pp. 4–12.

8. Colditz, Graham, et al., "Menopause and the Risk of Coronary Heart Disease in Women," *The New England Journal of Medicine* (April 30, 1987), 316:18, pp.1105–10.

9. "Consensus Development Conference: Prophylaxis and Treatment of Osteoporosis," *British Medical Journal* (October 10, 1987), 295, pp. 914–15.

10. Criqui, Michael H., et al., "Postmenopausal Estrogen Use and Mortality: Results from a Prospective Study in a Defined, Homogeneous Community," *American Journal of Epidemiology* (September 1988), 128:3, pp. 606–13.

11. Davis, Lisa, et al., "Tracking Women's Bone Loss," *In Health* (May/June 1990), 4:3, p. 11.

12. Dennerstein, Lorraine, "Depression in the Menopause," *Obstetrics and Gynecology Clinics of North America* (March 1987), 4:1, pp. 33–40.

13. Drinkwater, B.L., et al., "Bone Mineral Content of Amenorrheic and Eumenorrheic Athletes," *New England Journal of Medicine* (August 2, 1984), 311:5, pp. 277-81.

14. "Eating to Lower Your High Blood Cholesterol," NIH Publication No. 87-2920, U.S. Department of Health and Human Services, Washington, DC, September 1987.

15. Ettinger, Bruce, "Overview of the Efficacy of Hormonal Replacement Therapy," *American Journal of Obstetrics and Gynecology* (May 1987), 156:5, pp. 1298–1301.

16. Fahraeus, Lars, "The Effects of Estradiol on Blood Lipids and Lipoproteins in Postmenopausal Women," *Obstetrics and Gynecology* (November 1988), 72:5, pp. 18S-22S.

17. Gambrell, R. Don, "Estrogen-Progestogen Therapy During Menopause: Renewed Interest in the 1980s," *Postgraduate Medicine* (November 1, 1986), 80:6, pp. 261–7.

18. Genant, H. K., Cann, C, E., Ettinger, B., and Gordon, G. S., "Quanitative Computerized Tomography of Vertebral Spongiosa: A Sensitive Method for Detecting Early Bone Loss after Oophorectomy," *Annals of Internal Medicine* (1982), 97, pp. 699–705.

19. Gifford-Jones, W., *What Every Woman Should Know about Hysterectomy* (New York: Funk & Wagnell, 1977), p. 156–7.

20. Gould, Dinah, "Hidden Problems after a Hysterectomy," *Nursing Times* (June 4, 1986), pp. 43–6.

21. Greenblatt, Robert B., "The Use of Androgens in the Menopause and Other Gynecic Disorders," *Obstetrics and Gynecology Clinics of North America* (March 1987), 14:1, pp. 251–67.

22. Hillner, Bruce, Hollenberg, James P., and Pauker, Stephen G., "Postmenopausal Estrogens in the Prevention of Osteoporosis: Benefit Virtually Without Risk if Cardiovascular Effects Are Considered,"*American Journal of Medicine* (June 1986), 80:6, p. 1115.

23. Hreshchyshyn, Myroslaw, et al., "Effects of Natural Menopause, Hysterectomy, and Oophorectomy on Lumbar Spine and Femoral Neck Bone Densities," *Obstetrics and Gynecology* (October 1988), 72:4, pp. 631–7.

24. Jensen, Jytte and Christiansen, Claus, "Effects of Smoking on Serum Lipoproteins and Bone Mineral Content During Postmenopausal Hormone Replacement Therapy," *American Journal of Obstetrics and Gynecology* (October 1988), 159:4, pp. 820–5.

25. Judd, Howard and Utian, Wulf, "Current Perspectives in the Management of the Menopausal and Postmenopausal Patient," *American Journal of Obstetrics and Gynecology* (May 1987), 156:5, pp. 1279–1356.

26. Judd, Howard, "Efficacy of Transdermal Estradiol," *Obstetrics and Gynecology* (May 1987), 156, pp.1326–31.

27. Kiel, Douglas P., et al., "Hip Fracture and the Use of Estrogens in Postmenopausal Women: The Framingham Study," *New England Journal of Medicine* (November 5, 1987), 317:19, pp. 1169–74.

28. Knopp, Robert H., "The Effects of Postmenopausal Estrogen Therapy on the Incidence of Arteriosclerotic Vascular Disease," *Obstetrics and Gynecology* (November 1988), 72:5, pp. 23S–30S.

29. Lalinec-Michaud, M. and Engelsmann, F., "Anxiety, Fears and Depression Related to Hysterectomy," *Canadian Journal of Psychiatry* (February 1985), 30, pp. 44–7.

30. Lalinec-Michaud, Martine, et al., "Depression After Hysterectomy," *Psychosomatics* (Summer 1988), 29:3, pp. 307–13.

31. Lalinec-Michaud, Martine and Engelsmann, Frank, "Depression and Hysterectomy: A Prospective Study," *Psychosomatics* (July 1984), 25:7, pp. 550–8.

32. Lievertz, Randolph W., "Pharmacokinetics of Estrogens," *American Journal of Obstetrics and Gynecology* (May 1987), 156:5, pp. 1289–93.

33. Lindemann, E., "Observations on Psychiatric Sequelae to Surgical Operations on Women," *American Journal of Psychiatry* (1941), 98, pp. 132–7.

34. Lindsay, Robert, "Estrogen Therapy in the Prevention and Management of Osteoporosis," *American Journal of Obstetrics and Gynecology* (May 1987), 156:5, pp. 1347–51.

35. Lindsay, Robert, "Managing Osteoporosis: Current Trends, Future Possibilities," *Geriatrics* (March 1987), 42:3, pp. 35–40.

36. Lufkin, Edward, et al., "Estrogen Replacement Therapy: Current Recommendations," *Mayo Clinic Proceedings* (May 1988), 63, pp. 453–60.

37. Mack, T. M., et al., "Estrogens and Endometrial Cancer in a Retirement Community," *New England Journal of Medicine* (June 3, 1976), 294:23, pp. 1262–7.

38. Marcus, R., et al., "Menstrual Function and Bone Mass in Elite Women Distance Runners," *Annals of Internal Medicine* (February 1985), 102:2, pp. 158-63.

39. Morgan, Susanne, *Coping With a Hysterectomy: Your Own Choice, Your Own Solutions* (New York: Dial, 1982), p. 148.

40. Nachtigall, Lila E., "Cardiovascular Disease and Hypertension in Older Women," *Obstetrics and Gynecology Clinics of North America* (March 1987), 14:1, pp. 89–103.

41. Notelovitz, Morris, "Climacteric Medicine: Cornerstone for Midlife Health and Wellness," *Public Health Reports Supplement* (July/August 1986), pp. 116–23.

42. Notelovitz, Morris, "Exercise, Nurtrition, and the Coagulation Effects of Estrogen Replacement on Cardiovascular Health," *Obstetrics and Gynecology Clinics of North America* (March 1987), 14:1, pp. 121–39.

43. Pogrund, Hyman, Bloom, Ronald A., and Menczel, Jacob, "Preventing Osteoporosis: Current Practices and Problems," *Geriatrics* (May 1986), 41:5, pp. 55–71.

44. Rebar, Robert and Spitzer, Ilene, "The Physiology and Measurement of Hot Flushes," *American Journal of Obstetrics and Gynecology* (May 1987), 156:5, pp. 1284–7.

45. Reeve, J., et al., "Anabolic Effect of Human Parathyroid Hormone Fragment on Trabecular Bone Involutional Osteoporosis: A Multicenter Trial," *British Medical Journal* (June 7, 1984), 280:6228, pp 1340–4.

46. Richards, D. H., "A Post-Hysterectomy Syndrome," *The Lancet* (October 26, 1974), 2:7887, pp. 983–5.

47. Riggs, B. Lawrence, "Pathogenesis of Osteoporosis," *American Journal of Obstetrics and Gynecology* (May 1987), 156:5, pp. 1342–6.

48. Rivlin, Richard S., "Osteoporosis: Nutrition," *Public Health Reports Supplement* (July/August 1986), pp. 131–6.

49. Sarrel, Philip M., "Estrogen Replacement Therapy," *Obstetrics and Gynecology* (November 1988), 72:5, pp. 2S–5S.

50. Sarrel, Philip M., "Sexuality in the Middle Years," *Obstetrics and Gynecology Clinics of North America* (March 1987), 14:1, pp. 49–61.

51. Sobel, Solomon, "Osteoporosis: Regulatory View," *Public Health Reports Supplement* (July/August 1986), pp. 136–9.

52. Stampfer, Meir J., et al., "A Prospective Study of Postmenopausal Estrogen Therapy and Coronary Heart Disease," *New England Journal of Medicine* (October 24, 1985), 313:17, pp. 1044–8.

53. Steinberg, Karen K., "Women's Health: Osteoporosis—Introductory Remarks," *Public Health Reports Supplement* (July/August 1986), pp. 125–7.

54. Teran, Ana-Zully, Greenblatt, Robert B., and Chaddha, Jaswant S., "Changes in Lipoproteins with Various Sex Steroids," *Obstetrics and Gynecology Clinics of North America* (March 1987), 14:1, pp. 107–17.

55. Utian, Wulf H., "The Fate of the Untreated Menopause," *Obstetrics and Gynecology Clinics of North America* (March 1987), 14:1, pp. 1–11.

56. Utian, Wulf H., "Transdermal Estradiol Overall Safety Profile," *American Journal of Obstetrics and Gynecology* (1987), 156, pp. 1335–8.

57. Watts, Nelson B., "Osteoporosis," *American Family Physician* (November 1988), 38:5, pp. 193–205.

58. Watts, Nelson B., et al., "Intermittent Cyclical Etindronate Treatment of Postmenopausal Osteoporosis," *New England Journal of Medicine* (July 12, 1990), 323:2, pp. 73-9.

59. Webb, Christine and Wilson-Barnett, Jenifer, "Hysterectomy: Dispelling the Myths—Part I and II," *Nursing Times* (November 23/30, 1983), pp. 44–6, 52–4.

60. Wigfall-Williams, Wanda, *Hysterectomy: Learning the Facts, Coping with the Feelings, Facing the Future* (New York: Kesend, 1986), p. 49.

61. Wilson, Peter W. F., Garrison, Robert J., and Castelli, William P., "Postmenopausal Estrogen Use, Cigarette Smoking, and Cardiovascular Morbidity in Women Over 50: The Framingham Study," *New England Journal of Medicine* (October 24, 1985), 313:17, pp. 1038–43.

62. Youngs, David D. and Ehrhardt, Anke A., *Psychosomatic Obstetrics and Gynecology* (New York: Appleton-Century-Crofts, 1980), pp. 255–64.

63. Ziel, H. K. and Finkle, W. D., "Increased Risk of Endometrial Carcinoma among Users of Conjugated Estrogens," *New England Journal of Medicine* (December 4, 1975), 293:23, pp. 1167–70.

Chapter Nine

1. American College of Obstetricians and Gynecologists, "Estrogen Replacement Therapy," *ACOG Technical Bulletin* (April 1986), 93, pp. 1–5.

2. American College of Obstetricians and Gynecologists, "Prophylactic Oophorectomy," *ACOG Technical Bulletin* (December 1987), 111, pp. 1–5.

3. Armstrong, Bruce K., "Oestrogen Therapy After the Menopause—Boon or Bane?" *The Medical Journal of Australia* (March 7, 1988), 148, pp. 213–14.

4. Barrett-Conner, Elizabeth, "Postmenopausal Estrogen Replacement and Breast Cancer," *The New England Journal of Medicine* (August 3, 1989), 321:5, pp. 319–20.

5. Brinton, L. A., Hoover, R., and Fraumeni, J. F., "Menopausal Oestrogens and Breast Cancer Risk: An Expanded Case-Control Study," *British Journal of Cancer* (November 1986), 54:5, pp. 825–32.

6. Buring, J. E., et al., "A Prospective Cohort Study of Postmenopausal Hormone Use and Risk of Breast Cancer in U.S. Women," *American Journal of Epidemiology* (June 1987), 125:6, pp. 939–47.

7. Ernster, Virginia and Cummings, Steven, "Progesterone and Breast Cancer," *Obstetrics and Gynecology* (November 1986), 68:5, pp. 715–17.

8. Gambrell, R. Don, Maier, Robert C. and Sanders, Barbara I., "Decreased Incidence of Breast Cancer in Postmenopausal Estrogen-Progestogen Users," *Obstetrics and Gynecology* (October 1983), 62:4, pp. 435-43.

9. Gambrell, R. Don, "Use of Progestogen Therapy," *American Journal of Obstetrics and Gynecology* (May 1987), 156:5, pp. 1304–13.

10. Hillner, Bruce E., Hollenberg, James R., and Pauker, Stephen G., "Postmenopausal Estrogens in Prevention of Osteoporosis: Benefit Virtually Without Risk if Cardiovascular Effects Are Considered," *The American Jornal of Medicine* (June 1986), 80:6, p. 1115.

11. Horwitz, Ralph I., "Estrogens and Endometrial Cancer: Responses to Arguments and Current Status of an Epidemiologic Controversy," *The American Journal of Medicine* (September 1986) 81:3, pp. 503–7.

12. Hulka, Barbara S., "Replacement Estrogens and Risk of Gynecologic Cancers and Breast Cancer," *Cancer* (October 15, 1987), 60:8, pp. 1960–4.

13. Judd, Howard, "Efficacy of Transdermal Estradiol," *American Journal of Obstetrics and Gynecology* (May 1987), 156, pp. 1326–31.

14. Key, T. J. A. and Pike, M. C., "The Dose-Effect Relationship Between 'Unopposed' Oestrogens and Endometrial Mitotic Rate: Its Central Role in Explaining and Predicting Endometrial Cancer Risk," *British Journal of Cancer* (February 1988), 57:2, pp. 205–12.

15. Lufkin, Edward G., et al., "Estrogen Replacement Therapy: Current Recommendations," *Mayo Clinic Proceedings* (May 1988), 63, pp. 453–60.

16. Rohan, Thomas E. and McMichael, Anthony J., "Non-Contraceptive Exogenous Oestrogen Therapy and Breast Cancer," *The Medical Journal of Australia* (March 7, 1988), 148, pp. 217–21.

17. Shapiro, Samuel, et al., "Risk of Localized and Widespread Endometrial Cancer in Relation to Recent and Discontinued Use of Conjugated Estrogens," *New England Journal of Medicine* (October 17, 1985), 313:16, pp. 969–72.

18. Utian, Wulf H., "Transdermal Estradiol Overall Safety Profile," *American Journal of Obstetrics and Gynecology* (May 1987), 156:5, pp. 1335–8.

19. Whitehead, Malcolm I. and Fraser, David, "Controversies Concerning the Safety of Estrogen Replacement Therapy," *American Journal of Obstetrics and Gynecology* (May 1987), 156:5, pp. 1313–22.

20. Wingo, Phyllis A., et al., "The Risk of Breast Cancer in Post-menopausal Women Who Have Used Estrogen Replacement Therapy," *Journal of the American Medical Association* (January 9, 1987), 257:2, pp. 209–15.

Epilogue

1. Evans, Bergen, ed., *Dictionary of Quotations* (New York: Avelen, 1978), p. 94.

2. Llewellyn-Jones, Derek, *Everywoman: A Gynaecological Guide for Life* (London: Faber and Faber, 1971).

3. Scully, Diane, *Men Who Control Women's Health: The Miseducation of Obstetrician-Gynecologists* (Boston: Houghton Mifflin, 1980).

Sources

Figures

2.1. Syntex Laboratories, Inc., Palo Alto, CA., Copyright 1985.

3.1. Kistner, Robert, *Gynecology: Principles and Practice*, 4th ed., (Chicago: Year Book Medical Publishers, 1986), p. 197.

3.2. Kistner, Robert, *Gynecology: Principles and Practices*, 4th ed., (Chicago: Year Book Medical Publishers, 1986), p. 203.

3.3 Richard Wolf Medical Instruments Corporation, Rosemont, Illinois.

3.4 LaserSonics.

4.1 Richard Wolf Medical Instruments Corporation, Rosemont, Illinois.

4.2. Copyright 1988. Reprinted with permission of the American Fertility Society.

4.3. Copyright 1988. Reprinted with permission of the American Fertility Society.

4.4. Copyright 1988. Reprinted with permission of the American Fertility Society.

4.5. From: The American Fertility Society: Revised American Fertility Society Classification of Endometriosis: 1985. Fertil. Steril. 43:351, 1985. Reproduced with permission of the publisher, The American Fertility Society.

7.2. Wyeth-Ayerst Laboratories.

8.1. Sarrel, Philip, "Estrogen Replacement Therapy," *Obstetrics and Gynecology* (1988), 72:5, p. 3S.

8.3. Sarrel, Philip, "Estrogen Replacement Therapy," *Obstetrics and Gynecology* (1988), 72:5, p. 3S.

Figures 2.2, 2.3, 2.4, 7.1, 8.2, and 9.1 are original drawings by Brian Pendley.

Tables

1.1. "Hysterectomies in the United States: 1965–1984, *Vital and Health Statistics*, U.S. Department of Health and Human Services, National Health Survey, Series 13, No. 92.

4.1. The American Fertility Society: Revised American Fertility Society Classification of Endometriosis: 1985. Fertil. Steril. 43:351, 1985.

Droegmueller, William, Comprehensive Gynecology, (Washington, DC.: Mosby, 1987), p.501.

6.1. American Cancer Society, "Cancer Facts & Figures—1990" (1990), pp. 10–11.

American Cancer Society, *A Cancer Source Book for Nurses* (1981), pp. 79–86.

Barber, Hugh, *Manual of Gynecologic Oncology* (Philadelphia: Lippencott, 1989).

Petrek, Jeanne, *A Woman's Guide to the Prevention, Detection and Treatment of Cancer* (New York: McMillan, 1985), pp. 34–92.

Sidebars

Not All Cholesterol Is Created Equal

"Eating to Lower Your High Blood Cholesterol," NIH Publication No. 87-2920, U.S. Department of Health and Human Services, Washington, D.C., September, 1987.

Depression: A Self-Help Guide

American Psychiatric Association: *Diagnostic and Statistical Manual of Mental Disorders, Third Edition, Revised,* Washington, D.C., American Psychiatric Association, 1987.

Appendix B

Calcium Content in Milligram of Selected Foods

McIlwain, Harris H., et al., *Osteoporosis: Prevention, Management, Treatment* (New York: Wiley, 1988), pp. 101–15.

The First Step in Eating Right Is Buying Right

"Eating to Lower Your High Blood Cholesterol," NIH Publication No. 89-2920, U.S. Department of Health and Human Services, National Heart, Lung, and Blood Institute, Washington DC, June, 1989.

Quoted Materials

The quotations appearing on pages 2, 39, and 47 are reprinted by permission of Random House, Inc. and Alfred A. Knopf, Inc. from: *A Woman in Residence* by Michelle Harrison, M.D., Copyright © 1982.

The quotations appearing on pages ix, 10, and 11 are reprinted by permission of Walker and Company from: *Understanding Hysterectomy: A Woman's Guide* by F. G. Giustini and F.J. Feefer, Copyright © 1979.

The quotation appearing on pages 21-22 is excerpted from material originally appearing in the *New England Journal of Medicine* as "Elective Hysterectomy: Pro and Con" by John P. Bunker, M.D., volume 295, page 264, 1976.

The quotation appearing on page 25 is excerpted from material originally appearing in *The Journal of the American Medical Association* as "Prophylactic Hysterectomy at Oophorectomy in Young Women" by Paul G. Stumpf, M.D., volume 252, p. 1129, Copyright © 1984 by the American Medical Association.

The quotation appearing on page 67 is reprinted with permission of Charles Scribner's Sons, an imprint of MacMillan Publishing Company from: *Endometriosis* by Julia Older, Copyright © 1984 Julia Older.

The quotations appearing on pages 97 and 185 are reprinted by permission of Butterworth and Company (Publishers) Ltd. from: *Jeffcoate's Principles of Gynaecology* by Sir Norman Jeffcoate, Copyright © 1987.

The quotation appearing on pages 137-138 is reprinted by permission of The Putnam Publishing Group from: *NO MORE HOT FLASHES AND OTHER GOOD NEWS* by Penny Wise Budoff, M.D., Copyright © 1983 by Penny Wise Budoff, M.D.

The quotation appearing on page 139 is reprinted by permission of Michael Kesend Publishing, Ltd. 1025 Fifth Avenue, New York, New York 10028 from: *Hysterectomy: Learning the Facts, Coping with the Feelings, Facing the Future* by Wanda Wigfall-Williams, Copyright © 1986.

The quotation appearing on page 152 is excerpted from material originally appearing in *British Medical Journal* as "Consensus Development Conference: Prophylaxis and Treatment of Osteoporosis," volume 295, page 914, 1987.

The quotation appearing on page 200 is excerpted from material originally appearing in the *New England Journal of Medicine* as "Post-menopausal Estrogen Replacement and Breast Cancer" by Elizabeth Barrett-Conner, M.D., volume 321, page 320, 1989.

The quotation appearing on page 201 is reprinted by permission of Faber and Faber Limited Publishers from: *EVERYWOMAN: A GYNAECOLOGICAL GUIDE FOR LIFE* by Derek Llewellyn Jones, Copyright © 1971.

Glossary

A

Ablation. Removal or eradication, as by cutting or burning. (For example, *endometrial ablation*: the removal of the lining of the uterus by laser vaporization.)

Adenomyosis. Abnormal growth of the lining of the uterus so as to invade the muscular layer. Also called *internal endometriosis.*

Adhesion. A band of fibrous tissue that sometimes arises abnormally as a result of disease or surgery, thus causing the joining of structures that are not normally bound together.

Adnexa. A collective term for the ovaries, fallopian tubes, and uterine ligaments.

Adrenal Gland. A small organ located near the kidney and responsible for production of certain sex hormones, including testosterone and small amounts of estrogen.

Analgesic. A pain reliever.

Androgen. Male sex hormone.

Anovulatory. Lacking the release of an egg or "ovum" from the ovary.

Arteriosclerosis (Atherosclerosis). A condition in which deposits of cholesterol and other materials form within blood vessels, thus narrowing their diameters; also called "hardening of the arteries."

Atrophic Vaginitis. A type of vaginal irritation caused by the depletion of estrogen associated with menopause.

Atrophy. Wasting away or shrinking in size.

B

Beta Endorphin. A chemical substance produced by the body that naturally reduces pain and increases a sense of well-being.

Bilateral Tubal Ligation. A sterilization procedure during which the fallopian tubes are clamped, tied, or cut to obstruct the union of sperm and egg.

Biopsy. The removal of a sample of tissue for diagnostic examination. (For example, endometrial biopsy: the suctioning out and microscopic evaluation of the uterine lining.)

C

Calcitonin. A hormone produced by the thyroid gland that is responsible for maintaining calcium balance in the body, specifically by preventing its loss from bone.

Carcinoma. Cancer.

Castration. The act of rendering a man or woman incapable of reproducing by removing or destroying his or her sex organs; specifically, in a woman, her ovaries.

CAT Scan. Computerized Axial Tomography—a sophisticated type of X ray that uses computer analysis to generate an in-depth view of body tissues.

Cautery (cauterize; cauterization). A procedure used to destroy tissue by cold, heat, or chemicals.

Cervix. The lowermost portion of the uterus.

Chemotherapy. The use of drugs to treat various illnesses. (For example, in the case of cancer.)

Climacteric. Another word for menopause; that era in a woman's life when she may no longer bear children, said to begin once a woman has ceased to menstruate for one year.

Clitoris. A small structure located just outside the vagina and capable of erection during sexual arousal analagous to the penis.

Clitoridectomy. The surgical removal of the clitoris.

Colposcopy. A procedure using a magnifying lens to examine the cervix.

Cone Biopsy. The surgical removal of a cone-shaped area of the cervix for diagnostic and therapeutic purposes.

Corpus Luteum. The "yellow body" that is created from the follicle in the ovary once its egg has been released; responsible for the secretion of estrogen and progesterone.

Cryosurgery. The destruction of tissue via freezing.

Cul-de-sac. The pouch located behind the uterus.

Cystocele. A condition that arises when support structures weaken, allowing the bladder to drop down and protrude into the vagina.

D

D&C. *See* Dilation and Curettege.

Dilation and Curettage (D&C). A surgical procedure during which the cervix is stretched (dilation) to admit instruments that scrape and remove the lining of the uterus (curettage) for diagnostic and therapeutic purposes.

Dysfunctional Uterine Bleeding (DUB). Abnormal bleeding associated with hormonal imbalance.

Dysmenorrhea. Painful menstruation.

Dyspareunia. Pain during sexual intercourse.

E

Ectopic Pregnancy. The implantation of a fertilized egg outside of the uterus, almost always within the fallopian tube.

Endocrine. Pertaining to the system of organs in the body that produce chemical substances, called "hormones" that then exert their effects on other parts of the body.

Endometrial Ablation. *See* Ablation.

Endometrioma. A large mass containing endometrial tissue.

Endometriosis. A condition whereby tissue normally found only lining the uterus is present in abnormal locations throughout the body.

Endometrium. The tissue comprising the lining of the uterus.

Epithelium. The cells that cover the internal and external surfaces of the body.

Estrogen. The female sex hormone produced by the ovary and the adrenal gland which is responsible for the development of the fem-inizing characteristics of women as well as playing a role in the menstrual cycle and in pregnancy. Three types are naturally produced by the body: estradiol, estrone, and estriol.

F

Fallopian Tubes. The structures located between the uterus and ovaries responsible for the transport of the egg. Also called the oviducts.

Fibroid. A noncancerous tumor comprised of uterine muscle tissue. There are three types: serosal, intramural, and submucous. Also called a leiomyoma or myoma.

Follicle. Receptacles within the ovary that house immature eggs.

Follicle Stimulating Hormone (FSH). Causes the maturation and release of one egg each month from the ovarian follicles.

G

Gonadotrophin Releasing Factors/Hormones (GnRH). Substances having a stimulating effect on the sex hormones.

H

Hemorrhage. Bleeding.

Homeostasis. The maintenance of a stable, normal, and balanced body system or internal environment through a system of feedback controls and checks and balances.

Hormone. A chemical produced at one site in the body which is responsible for the actions of an organ at another site.

Human Chorionic Gonadotrophin (HCG). The hormone responsible for maintaining estrogen and progesterone levels during pregnancy until the placenta takes over.

Hyperplasia. The growth of normal cells in abnormally large numbers. (For example, endometrial hyperplasia: the overgrowth of the uterine lining under the influences of prolonged estrogen exposure.)

Hypertrophy. The enlargement of a structure due to an increase in the size of its cells.

Hypothalamus. A structure in the brain responsible for maintaining body temperature, for mediating sleep and feeding, and for the release of hormones regulating the menstrual cycle.

Hysterectomy. The surgical removal of the uterus; variations include: subtotal, total, radical, abdominal, and vaginal.

Hysteroscopy. A diagnostic test during which a fiberoptic scope is introduced into the body via the cervix to examine the uterus.

I

In Vitro Fertilization. The union of sperm and egg outside of the body. Also called test tube babies.

Incontinence. The inability to consciously control urination or defecation. (For example, stress incontinence: leakage of urine during laughter, coughing, or straining.)

Infertility. The inability to conceive after one year of unprotected intercourse.

Internal Endometriosis. See Adenomyosis.

L

Labia Majora/Minora. The large and small outer and inner lips located at the entrance to the vagina.

Laminaria. Rods of sterilized seaweed inserted into the cervix to dilate it, thus facilitating certain procedures, such as vaginal myomectomies.

Laparoscopy. A diagnostic test during which a fiberoptic scope is inserted through the navel to view the internal pelvic organs.

Laparotomy. The term for open abdominal surgery.

Laser. Light amplification by stimulated emission of radiation—a device which transforms light into an intense and highly focused beam capable of generating heat that can cut, coagulate, or vaporize tissue. Types discussed in this book include the "ND:YAG," "Argon," "KTP," and "CO_2" lasers.

Leiomyoma. See Fibroid.

Libido. Sex drive.

Luteinizing Hormone (LH). A chemical that facilitates the conversion of a follicle to a corpus luteum.

Lymph. A fluid that bathes tissues and is responsible for the transport of certain substances throughout the body.

M

Malignancy. A tendency to progress in severity, often resulting in death, as in cancer.

Mammogram. A specialized X ray taken of the breasts to screen for cancer and other pathology.

Menarche. The term used for the onset of menstruation.

Menopause. See Climacteric.

Menstruation. The monthly cycle of hormone production and ovarian activities that prepares the female body for pregnancy, culminating in shedding of the uterine lining and bleeding if conception does not take place.

Metabolism. The sum of all activities that sustain life, including those that result in creation of body structures as well as those resulting in tissue destruction with the subsequent release of energy. The rate at which we burn energy is called our metabolic rate.

Metastasis. The spread of disease from one organ to another, as in cancer metastasis.

Mons pubis. The fleshy mound of tissue convering the pubic bone in women.

Morbidity/Mortality. Pertaining to disease/death, respectively.

MRI. Magnetic resonance imaging—a high-tech diagnostic test utilizing a powerful magnet and a computer to analyze tissue structures.

Multiparity. The condition of having had more than one child.

Myoma. See Fibroid.

Myomectomy. The surgical excision of uterine fibroids.

Myometrium. The muscular, middle layer of the uterus.

N

Neonatal. Pertaining to the newborn.

Neoplasia. Pertaining to the abnormal and uncontrollable growth of tissue, as in cancer.

O

Oophorectomy. The surgical removal of the ovary.

Os. The opening of the cervix.

Osteoporosis. A condition where bone weakens and deteriorates as a result of bone destruction exceeding production.

Ovary. The organ that produces and houses the female reproductive cells, called ova. It is also the site of estrogen and progesterone production.

Oviducts. See Fallopian Tubes.

Ovulation. The monthly release of an egg from the ovary that will either be followed by pregnancy, if a sperm cell is present to join with it, or menstruation, if conception does not occur.

Ovum (Ova). The egg or female reproductive cell.

P

Pap Smear. A screening test for cervical cancer performed by scraping the superficial cells from the cervix during a pelvic examination and subjecting them to laboratory analysis for abnormalities.

Parathyroid Gland. Four small bodies located in the neck and responsible for maintaining calcium balance.

Pelvic Inflammatory Disease (PID). An infection, usually sexually transmitted, involving the uterus, ovaries, and/or fallopian tubes.

Perineum. The floor of the pelvis. The region located between the pubic bone and the anus.

Pituitary Gland. A pea-sized organ within the brain, responsible for regulating hormones associated with the menstrual cycle. It works in conjunction with the hypothalamus.

Placenta. A structure created within the uterus during pregnancy that links the mother's circulation to the developing fetus's, and serves as a source of nutrition and waste elimination.

Polyp. A noncancerous, protruding growth. (For example, cervical polyp.)

Postpartum. The period immediately after childbirth.

Progesterone/Progestin. A hormone produced in the ovary, adrenal gland, and placenta (of a pregnant woman) that prepares for and sustains pregnancy.

Prolapse. The dropping down of an organ into an abnormal location as a result of a weakening of the support structures that normally hold it in place.

Proliferative Phase. The stage of the menstrual cycle when the uterine lining is being built up in preparation for pregnancy.

Prophylactic. Preventative.

Prostaglandin. A chemical carrying out several functions in the body, including the initiation of uterine contractions, which causes menstrual cramps in some women.

R

Radiotherapy. The use of potent X rays to destroy abnormal tissue, as in the treatment of cancer.

Rectocele. A condition that arises when support structures weaken, allowing the rectum to prolapse into the vagina.

Resectoscope. A surgical device that is inserted into the uterus and used to remove tissue there for diagnostic and/or therapeutic purposes.

S

Salpingitis. Infection and inflammation of the fallopian tubes.

Salpingo-Oophorectomy. The surgical removal of the ovaries and fallopian tubes.

Sarcoma. A cancerous tumor. (For example, leiomyosarcoma—a cancerous fibroid.)

Secretory (Luteal) Phase. The phase of the menstrual cycle following formation of the corpus luteum and progesterone release.

Smegma. A cheesy discharge, made up of cellular debris and found in the vaginal area.

Sonogram. A diagnostic test utilizing sound waves to detect differences in tissue densities and thus to analyze body organs.

Speculum. A plastic or metal device inserted during a pelvic exam to separate the walls of the vagina, allowing a clearer view of the cervix.

Steroids. A group of substances of a similar chemical structure. This family includes the sex hormones.

T

Testosterone. The male sex hormone responsible for the development of masculinizing characteristics.

Thrombophlebitis. A condition in which a blood clot forms within a vein, leading to its inflammation; results in pain and impaired circulation.

Toxic Shock Syndrome. A potentially fatal bacterial infection usually occurring in menstruating women using tampons and marked by high fever, vomiting, diarrhea, rash, dizziness, sore throat, and other flulike symptoms.

Transdermal. Across the skin; as in transdermal estrogen patches—a type of patch that is applied to the skin allowing the systematic release of estrogen into the body through skin penetration.

Transformation/Transitional Zone. An area of the cervix bordering two types of cells and highly susceptible to cervical cancer.

Tumor. An abnormal growth of tissue that may or may not be cancerous.

U

Ultrasound. See Sonogram.

Uterus. The organ of the body within which a fetus develops. It may have other functions that have yet to be clarified by scientists.

Index

A

Abdominal hysterectomy, 188–189
Ablation, 91,247
Abnormal corpus luteum, 99
Adenomatous hyperplasia, 113
Adenomyosis
    definition, 68,94,247
    dysmenorrhea, 94
Adhesions, 72,85,247
Adnexa, 247
Adolescent endometriosis, 89
Adrenal gland, 247
Agonists, 55–56
Alcohol, 154
Analgesic, 247
Androgen, 29,33,57,103,247
Angina pectoris, 162
Anorexia nervosa, 151
Anovulatory bleeding, 99–100,247
Anti-estrogens, 56–57,93
Anti-inflammatory medication, 57
Antigen, 88
Antiprogesterones, 56
Antiprostaglandins, 103
Anxiety, 167
Argon laser, 58,91
Arteriosclerosis, 160–162,247
Atrophic vaginitis, 37,144,247
Atrophy, 247
Atypia *see:* Inflammation

B

Basal cells, 108
Benign breast disease, 196

Beta endorphins, 34,175,247
Bilateral tubal ligation, 247
Biopsy
    cone, 111
    definition, 248
    endometrial, 99,101,113,199
Birth control pills *see:* Oral
    contraceptives
Bladder prolapse, 127,145
Bladder symptoms, 145
Bleeding
    and endometriosis, 76
    abnormal uterine, 98,120,188
    anovulatory, 99–100
    dysfunctional uterine, 98,99
    from fibroids, 43–44
Blood-borne endometriosis, 72–73
Bone density, 150
Breast cancer, 122,195–196

C

Caffeine, 154
Calcitonin, 156,248
Calcium 125 *see* Serum Calcium 125
Calcium, 153
Cancer
    breast, 122,195–196
    cervix, 106–112,115
    definition, 106
    endometrial, 60,112–115,116,194
    endometrium, 122
    fallopian tubes, 119
    ovary, 116–119,122
    penile, 115
    statistics, 106